Towards the Prevention
of Cancer

Edited by

Amen Sibtain

Summaries   *nposium and*
the Jephco   *April 2007.*
These p   *on of the*
panelli   *ociety of*
Medicir   *bas been*

© 2007 Royal Society of Medicine Press Ltd

Published by the Royal Society of Medicine Press Ltd
1 Wimpole Street, London W1G 0AE, UK
Tel: +44 (0)20 7290 2921
Fax: +44 (0)20 7290 2929
Email: publishing@rsm.ac.uk
Website: www.rsmpress.co.uk

British Library Cataloguing in Publication Data
A catalogue record for this book is available from the British Library

ISBN 978-1-85315-796-7

Distribution in Europe and Rest of World:

Marston Book Services Ltd
PO Box 269
Abingdon
Oxon OX14 4YN, UK
Tel: +44 (0)1235 465500
Fax: +44 (0)1235 465555
Email: direct.order@marston.co.uk

Distribution in Australia and New Zealand:

Elsevier Australia
30–52 Smidmore Street
Marrickville NSW 2204, Australia
Tel: +61 2 9517 8999
Fax: +61 2 9517 2249
Email: service@elsevier.com.au

Distribution in the USA and Canada:

Royal Society of Medicine Press Ltd
c/o BookMasters Inc
30 Amberwood Parkway
Ashland, OH 44805, USA
Tel: +1 800 247 6553/+1 800 266 5564
Fax: +1 419 281 6883
Email: orders@bookmasters.com

Typeset by Phoenix Photosetting, Chatham, Kent

Printed in Great Britain by Bell & Bain, Glasgow, UK

Contents

Section Three: The Impact of Screening for Common Cancers

The Jephcott Lecture

Presenters and Participants

Professor Wendy Atkin
CANCER RESEARCH UK COLORECTAL UNIT, IMPERIAL COLLEGE LONDON, LONDON, UK

Professor Sir Leszek Borysiewicz
IMPERIAL COLLEGE LONDON, LONDON, UK

Dr Peter Boyle
INTERNATIONAL AGENCY FOR RESEARCH ON CANCER, LYON, FRANCE

Professor David Coggon
MRC EPIDEMIOLOGY RESOURCE CENTRE, UNIVERSITY OF SOUTHAMPTON, SOUTHAMPTON, UK

Professor Sir Alan Craft
DEPARTMENT OF CHILD HEALTH, ROYAL VICTORIA INFIRMARY, NEWCASTLE UPON TYNE, UK

Professor Paul Elliott
IMPERIAL COLLEGE LONDON, LONDON, UK

Dr Silvia Franceschi
INFECTIONS AND CANCER EPIDEMIOLOGY GROUP, INTERNATIONAL AGENCY FOR
RESEARCH ON CANCER, LYON, FRANCE

Professor the Baroness Finlay of Llandaff
PRESIDENT, ROYAL SOCIETY OF MEDICINE

Dr Michael Michell
BREAST RADIOLOGY DEPARTMENT, KING'S COLLEGE HOSPITAL NHS TRUST, LONDON, UK

Professor Alex Markham
CANCER RESEARCH UK

Professor Sir Richard Peto
CLINICAL TRIALS SERVICE UNIT, UNIVERSITY OF OXFORD, OXFORD, UK

Professor Bruce Ponder
CANCER RESEARCH UK CAMBRIDGE RESEARCH INSTITUTE, CAMBRIDGE, UK

Professor Elio Riboli
DEPARTMENT OF EPIDEMIOLOGY & PUBLIC HEALTH, IMPERIAL COLLEGE LONDON, LONDON, UK

Professor Mike Richards
NATIONAL CANCER DIRECTOR, LONDON, UK

Dr John Scadding
DEAN, ROYAL SOCIETY OF MEDICINE

Dr Amen Sibtain

DEPARTMENT OF CLINICAL ONCOLOGY/RADIOLOGY, ST BARTHOLOMEW'S HOSPITAL, LONDON, UK

Professor Stephen Spiro

DEPARTMENT OF THORACIC MEDICINE, UNIVERSITY COLLEGE HOSPITAL, LONDON, UK

Professor Robin Williamson

EMERITUS DEAN AND PRESIDENT-ELECT, ROYAL SOCIETY OF MEDICINE

Preface

Since 1959, a biennial lecture has been held at the Royal Society of Medicine in honour of Sir Harry Jephcott. In 2007, for the first time, a day-long symposium was arranged to complement the topic of the Jephcott Lecture. This publication represents the proceedings of this symposium.

Research on cancer leads to year-on-year improvements in treatment, but research in prevention of cancer is just as important, as is early detection, which leads to a greater likelihood of effective and curative treatment. Although much is still to be learned through research, great strides have already been made in understanding the cause of numerous cancers and in preventing cancers through a variety of approaches. Advances have been achieved through study of the genetic predisposition to certain cancers, epidemiological analysis and investigation of environmental factors that contribute to causation. The first half of the book examines these important topics. The second half focuses on early detection and screening for some common cancers, as well as considering the application of these approaches to cancer in children. The book finishes with the Jephcott Lecture on vaccine-based approaches to cancer prevention.

JOHN SCADDING
Dean, Royal Society of Medicine

Introduction

AMEN SIBTAIN

Prevention of disease is part of the fabric of medical philosophy. Preventing cancer avoids suffering and the acute and long-term side-effects of treatment, and is largely cost-effective. Advances in cancer prevention affect populations and so clearly save lives with broad brushstrokes of intelligent health policy rather than the 'pointillism' of cancer treatment.

The effectiveness and value of any policy or manoeuvre is enhanced when those at risk are targeted. For instance, being able to detect highly penetrant single-gene defects that cause early onset of cancer, guided by Mendelian inheritance patterns, identifies a group who would benefit from intervention or screening. However, inherited defects with small effects appear to work together to control genetic predisposition to late-onset epithelial cancers. This *polygenic variation* and its practical implications are discussed in the first chapter of this volume. The knowledge base required to refine screening stratagems based on the causative platform of interacting genetic mutations is enormous, and efforts to achieve this are underway.

Another obvious starting point in prevention is identifying the cause. The realm of possible causative agents is dynamic, varying in time and place. Unexpected local increases in cancer incidence, identified in cluster analysis studies, may highlight coincident exposure to a causative agent to reveal an association that drives a hypothesis. However, this surveillence as an early-warning system is only as good as the data that drive it, and lessons have been learnt from the Sellafield story. The second chapter recounts this and describes how these lessons have shaped the Small Area Health Statistics Unit.

Observational studies have been successful in identifying environmental and behavioural risk factors, the major culprits discussed in the following chapters. This knowledge informs health policy, health education, national legislation and individual choice. The European Prospective Investigation into Cancer and Nutrition has revealed fascinating and some surprising insights into the risk of cancer (e.g. the association between height and the risk of colorectal cancer), and has confirmed the complex multifactorial interactions between diet and malignancy.

Decades of evidence confirmed that smoking causes cancer, the number of deaths – premature deaths – is sobering. The description of this epidemiology by Sir Richard Peto illustrates the entirely preventable 450 million tobacco-related deaths that will happen if political will is lacking.

Infections are also associated with cancer development. Nearly one-fifth of all cancers worldwide are attributable to infection, providing a defined target for cancer prevention. Other environmental factors in the workplace, identified by well-coordinated scientific evaluation, have lead to the banning of asbestos and tight control on the industrial use of a variety of chemical carcinogens.

Despite epidemiological knowledge and the removal of causative factors, cancer still develops. Early detection aims to enhance cure rates, and less advanced disease requires less aggressive treatment with lower morbidity. In the UK, screening programmes in healthy 'at risk' populations are established for cancers of the breast, cervix and bowel, on the basis of evidence that lives are saved. Controversy still surrounds the screening of the other 'big' two – prostate and lung cancer – and perhaps the future lies in as-yet unidentified gene-based risk models. Studies of screening in paediatric cancer illustrate how occasionally prevention is not found to be worthwhile.

Vaccination, along with sanitation and antibiotics, has been the one of the greatest medical advances. Building on understanding of the role of human papillomavirus in cancer, a vaccine-based approach to the prevention of cervical cancer is now a reality. The final chapter in this volume explains the background and development of what will hopefully prove to be a breakthrough in the prevention of cancer.

The Towards the Prevention of Cancer symposium and the Jephcott Lecture, given by Professor Sir Leszek Borysiewicz, at the Royal Society of Medicine in 2007 were enormously successful. The topics covered were highly pertinent and the meeting brought together a group of internationally renowned leaders in the field. They have all contributed to this volume, resulting in a successful presentation of the scientific and practical aspects of the causation, prevention and early detection of malignancy.

Thanks are due to all the contributors, to the editorial team of the RSM Press, and to the President and Dean of the RSM for initiating an excellent symposium.

Section One: Taking a Broad View

Genetic predisposition to cancer

BRUCE PONDER

Introduction

In families with multiple cases of cancers, predisposition to breast and ovarian cancers due to inheritance of rare but strongly predisposing mutations in the *BRCA1* and *BRCA2* genes is well recognized. Any woman in such a family is at high risk, and if such a gene is known to be present, the family members can be offered genetic testing and counselling. If a woman is found not to have the gene, her risk of cancer is the same as in the population as a whole. If she has inherited one of the mutations, she has an 80% lifetime risk of cancer based on the gene's penetrance (the probability that the gene will be expressed as cancer by a given age). In Figure 1, woman A has a 50% chance of inheriting the gene mutation and an 80% lifetime risk of cancer if she has inherited the gene; her risk for breast cancer on the basis of these data alone would start to increase at the age of 30 years, reaching about 40% by the age of 80 years.[1]

The real-life situation is more complicated, however, as the woman's family history must be taken into account. For example, the risk of a 40-year-old woman with a *BRCA1* mutation having breast cancer by the age of 80 years is just less than 20%, but this decreases if there are no other women in the family with breast cancer and increases progressively the stronger the family history of other breast cancers. This is because penetrance of the *BRCA1* mutation is influenced by the genetic context in which it is being expressed – that is, the effects of multiple other genes. In multiple-case families, so-called 'modifying' genes can be presumed to be exerting a combined effect that increases the penetrance of the BRCA mutation. Modifiers that affect the risk attached to a *BRCA1* mutation might also be predisposing genes in their own right, and this gives rise to the idea of polygenic predisposition.

Polygenic predisposition[2]

Polygenic predisposition has very important implications for early detection and prevention that are likely to become of practical relevance in the next 10–20 years. It can be described, for example, in terms of the genetics of face shape. Every person's face is different not because people have mutations in single genes such as *BRCA1* but because we are all born with a set of normal genetic variants, the combination of which determines face shape. Polygenic variation also determines the risks of breast cancer, other cancers, hypertension, diabetes, asthma, etc. An overall measure of the influence of genetic predisposition for breast cancer can be estimated from the extent of family clustering. On average, a woman who has a relative affected by breast cancer has about a twofold increased risk compared with the population as a whole. Around 15–20% of genetic predisposition is explained by mutations in *BRCA1* and *BRCA2*

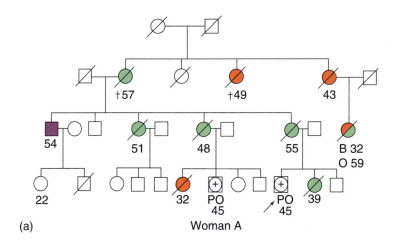

(a)   Woman A

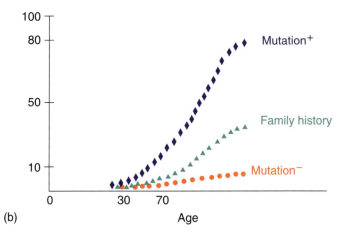

(b)   Age

Figure 1
A multiple-case breast and ovarian cancer family (b) and genetic prediction of risk in such a family (b).

and another 3–5% by rare mutations in other genes, but 75–80% of genetic predisposition is still to be explained (Figure 2). Although such rare, strongly predisposing '*BRCA*-like' genes may exist, they are likely to account for a only small number of cases, and data suggest a high proportion of cases will have a polygenic basis.[3]

Polygenic predisposition is important not because of the proportion of the total incidence of breast cancer it accounts for, however, but because of its effect on the distribution of risk in the population. From birth, some women will have a genetic profile that includes a large number of high-risk genetic variants, some will have only a few high-risk genetic variants and most will lie between the two extremes. The difference in risk between the two extremes determines the practical clinical significance of the risk: for example, a twofold difference between the top and bottom quintiles of risk is not significant, but a 30- or 40-fold difference

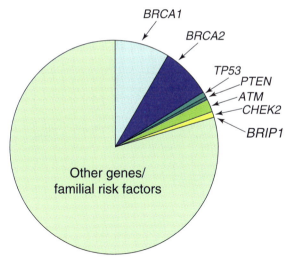

Figure 2
Susceptibility to breast cancer.

has potentially very important implications for the occurrence of a high proportion of breast cancer in a relatively small proportion of the population.

When a multiplicative genetic model was applied to the general East Anglian population around Cambridge, UK, Pharoah et al[4] found a 40-fold difference in risk between the top and bottom quintiles (Figure 3a). The distribution of risk in women destined to have breast cancer (a right-shifted curve because these women on average have a higher risk) predicted that half of all cases of breast cancer occur in the 12% of the distribution who are at greatest risk; conversely, of course, those at lowest risk have fewer cases of breast cancer. The inclusion of real numbers in this model rather than arbitrary risks allows the absolute risk of a woman developing breast cancer by the age of 70 years to be determined (Figure 3b). At the high-risk end of the distribution, 10% of the population have a risk of at least 12% by the age of 70, and this 10% of the population account for about 46% of all cases of breast cancer. Although the accuracy of this model is yet to be confirmed, it could be useful in selecting populations at higher or lower risk for studies of interventions. Similarly, at the low end of the risk spectrum, half of the population account for only 12% of breast cancer. As mammographic screening is believed to prevent about one-third of deaths from breast cancer, this knowledge could be used to argue that excluding the half of the population at lowest risk from the mammographic screening programme would result in 'only' an additional 4% of deaths from breast cancer, although this is controversial in terms of a whole plethora of social, ethical and legal issues.

The above estimates are based on the assumption that all predisposing gene mutations can be identified, but it is very unlikely that all of the culprit genes will be found and that the distribution will be defined completely. Figure 3(c) shows the risk distribution when only 50% of the genetic variation can be identified; although the degree of enrichment is less strong, it probably is still useful. It may thus be necessary to identify about half of the genes that contribute to the distribution in order for the model to be useful in practice. If the polygenic

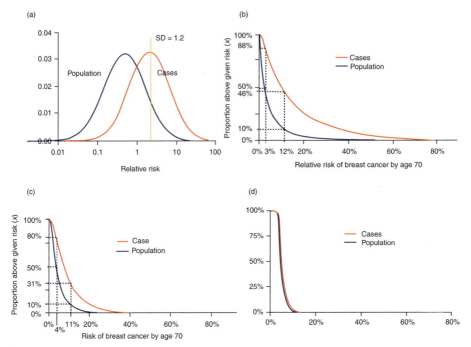

Figure 3

Model of risk distribution in breast cancer cases and controls from East Anglian Study using arbitrary log-scale of risks (a), proportion of population and cases above specified risk when 100% of genes scoreable using real-life numbers (b), individual risk prediction when 50% of genetic variation is scoreable (c) and proportion of population and cases above specified risk based on a widely used combination of clinical risk factors (d).

model is proved to be effective, it should provide a much stronger instrument for estimating risk than existing clinical risk tools. For example, women's risk of breast cancer is already stratified in the now classical Gail model on the basis of risk factors such as clinical findings, family history, benign breast disease and age, but although this model shows a difference between those at highest and lowest risk, almost no enrichment is present (Figure 3d).

Identifying genes

Identification of common weak genes in a population requires the use of a case–control design (or association study) rather than the linkage approach used to identify strong genes that segregate through families.[5] Such a design involves two groups: breast cancer cases and healthy controls from the same population. Researchers look for variants in the DNA sequence in candidate genes (genes plausibly thought to relate to breast cancer) that might affect the function or control of the gene and then determine whether those variants are more common in cases than in controls using single nucleotide polymorphisms (SNPs: single base variants in the DNA) as markers. If such variants are significantly and reproducibly more common in cases than controls, the inference is that those variants have an influence on breast cancer susceptibility.

This linkage disequilibrium (or association mapping) approach can be illustrated with the help of Figure 4(a). This might represent, for example, part of a DNA sequence from chromosome 6 (it might be part of the estrogen receptor) from an ancestor in Africa 100 000 years ago. At some point later, an adenosine (A) nucleotide in the sequence in one person's chromosome mutated to a guanosine (G), and in another individual a cytidine (C) mutated to a thymidine (T); as a result, the population then included three different versions of this chromosome. Some time later, the third chromosome underwent a further mutation – a change that produces a coding change in the estrogen receptor resulting in an alteration in its properties and a predisposition to breast cancer. Association mapping aims to compare the frequency of this functional change in the estrogen receptor in cases and controls to show that it is indeed the cause of breast cancer susceptibility.

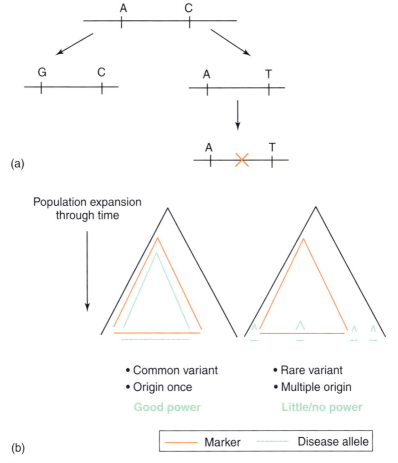

Figure 4
Schematic representation of the principles behind linkage disequilibrium (or association mapping) (a) and the dependence of association studies on genetic models (b).

The problem with all studies that seek to identify culprit genes is that the variant that leads to the change of function of the gene that predisposes to disease is generally unknown, which means that other sequence variants in the DNA such as SNPs have to be used as arbitrary markers. This requires a number of assumptions, and Figure 4(b), which shows a schematic representation of the history of a population expanding through tens of thousands of years, can be used to illustrate the most important of these. At some point in the depicted population, an SNP, which is used as a genetic marker, arose and expanded to some of the population over time, as indicated by the red line; the green lines represent the disease-causing variants being sought. If the variant and marker each arose only once and at about the same time in the history of population, they will subtend roughly equal segments of the current population and that marker will report efficiently and with good power on this disease gene. This is called the 'common variant common disease' hypothesis. Unfortunately, however, a different model might be operating, and researchers may be using a marker common in the population but searching for a disease gene that arose very recently and that would subtend only a tiny part of the population. Indeed, the gene might also contain multiple disease alleles that have arisen independently. In those situations, the marker has very poor power to identify the disease gene. More work is needed to elucidate this situation.

Undeterred, researchers in Cambridge set out to use the common variant common disease model, chose a number of genes and pathways that might be related to breast cancer, and selected common variants as markers so as to report as completely as possible on all other common variants in the gene. The study involved 4600 patients with invasive breast cancer from the East Anglian regional cancer registry who were 70 years or younger at diagnosis as cases, and 4600 women older than 50 years from the EPIC-Norfolk diet and cancer cohort as controls. These numbers were chosen to provide a sample size with the power to detect any variant that accounts for 1% of the total genetic effect. This study was funded for about 9 years by the Cancer Research Campaign and Cancer Research UK, during which time 200 genes were examined.

The top three provisional hits were in the estrogen receptor α gene (*ESR1*) ($p = 8 \times 10^{-5}$), the caspase 8 gene (*CASP8*) ($p = 1 \times 10^{-7}$) and the transforming growth factor β1 gene (*TGFB1*) ($p = 1 \times 10^{-4}$) (the *CASP8* observation was made in Sheffield and confirmed in Cambridge). Although these *p*-values seem convincing, in this situation it is a matter of prior probabilities: there is so much genome and so few genes are actually likely to be involved that strong statistical evidence is required to interpret anything as a real effect rather than chance. The hypothesis is that most of the many variants in the genome are neutral, some create a slight predisposition to breast cancer and a few are slightly protective. This means that most of the genetic effects are likely to be quite small, and there will be a problem in distinguishing true signals from statistical noise. The only way to circumvent this problem is to show that the results can be replicated in larger case–control sets. To do this, an international consortium has been set up, which now has 30 000 cases and 30 000 controls, to replicate potentially positive findings to prove they are real. Investigations with respect to the *ESR1* gene are being replicated at the time of writing, while the other two candidate genes have been confirmed as having real effects. The polymorphism in the *TGFB1* gene affects the signal peptide transforming growth factor β (TGF-β) and modifies secretion of the protein, which is probably the biological basis of its influence on breast cancer susceptibility.

Genome-wide association study

The genes thus far identified account for only a small proportion of the overall genetic contribution to breast cancer, and researchers ideally want to see if there is a smaller number of genes with larger effects: but because there will be very few such genes, looking for them one at a time is inefficient. The solution is a genome-wide association study, in which thousands of genes are examined in one experiment.[6] A study powered to look for common variants that explain 1% of the genetic effect thus began in 2003. Stage 1 started with 266 722 SNPs, which were designed to tag the whole genome as effectively as possible,[7] 400 cases from families at high risk of breast cancer but that were thought to lack the *BRCA1* or *BRCA2* mutations, and 400 women older than 50 years from the EPIC-Norfolk population as controls. Genotype frequencies were compared, and those with *p*-values >0.05 were discarded, while those with *p*-values <0.05 were carried through to stage 2 (about 12 000 (~5%) of the original SNPs). Stage 2 involved the 4600 cases and 4600 controls described earlier. Figure 5 summarizes the results from stage 2,[8] plotting the observed chi-squared values against the expected distribution. If no genetic effect was present, the expected and observed curves would overlay each other, but the observed line diverges upwards, which indicates the presence of a genetic effect. The divergence at the top end of the graph seems promising, but the divergence almost from the origin is worrying, as it is implausible that all of this reflects real genetic effect. The most likely explanation is the presence of some systematic bias in the study – either a hidden genetic structure in the population (population stratification) or a bias in genotyping between the case and control samples (genotyping bias). This was dealt with by using a correction factor for the initial difference in slope, and further studies were done to confirm that the differences at the top end of the curves were indeed reproducible and significant.

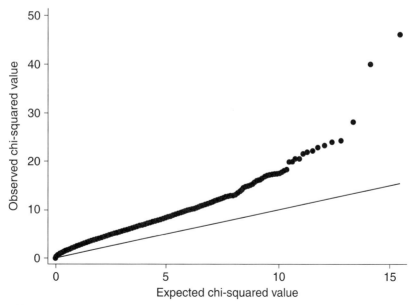

Figure 5
Observed versus expected distribution of chi-squared values in stage 2 of the genome-wide association study.

Table 1 *Summary of results after stages 1 and 2 of the genome-wide association study*

Level of significance	Observed	Observed adjusted	Expected
<0.00001	14	12	0.48
0.00001–0.0001	13	11	3.5
0.0001–0.001	103	88	57.3
0.001–0.01	509	463	342.2
0.01–0.05	1087	1005	939.7

Table 1 summarizes the results after stages 1 and 2 and shows a large excess, even after adjustment, in observed over expected findings. Whether this is a real effect or technical artefact is yet to be determined. The SNPs with p-values $>10^{-4}$ were discarded and those with p-values $<10^{-4}$ were taken into stage 3 of the study. This involved the international Breast Cancer Association Consortium (BCAC), which undertook 21 case–control studies in 21 668 cases involving invasive breast cancer, 967 cases of ductal carcinoma in situ, 20 973 controls and the top 30 SNPs from stages 1 and 2. Of these SNPs, six from five different loci (*FGFR2*, *TNRC9*, *MAP3K1*, *LSP1* and a 'gene desert' on chromosome 8q) showed consistent results, with a combined p-value across the whole study $<10^{-8}$, which is the current international standard. A further four SNPs had weak but consistent evidence, which suggests they have small effects that do not quite reach statistical significance. Finally, 20 SNPs were presumably statistical flukes in the first two stages, because they produced no evidence and the global p-value across all showed no significance. The top hits are discussed in more detail elsewhere.[8] The results from all collaborating groups around the world for the top 'hit', *FGFR2*, are shown in Figure 6; this highlights that the results were replicated consistently, with an overall p-value of 2×10^{-76} – powerful evidence of a real effect. Table 2 summarizes the characteristics of the top five hits.

The genome-wide study has been successful in finding common predisposing genes. Loci from the genome-wide and candidate studies so far explain about 5% of the overall genetic effect, although about 50% will probably need to be explained for results to be useful for prediction of breast cancer risk for individuals in the population. Most genes identified were novel for cancer susceptibility, were unlikely to have been considered previously and seem mostly to be regulatory rather than structural variants.

Table 2 *Best SNPs for each of the five top loci in the genome-wide association study*

Locus	Combined p-value trend	Allele frequency (%)	Attributable risk (%)	Genetic variance explained (%)
A	2×10^{-76}	38	16	2
B	1×10^{-36}	25	10	0.9
C	7×10^{-20}	28	9	0.5
D	5×10^{-12}	40	4	0.1
D	3×10^{-9}	30	4	0.1
			Variance explained	3.6%

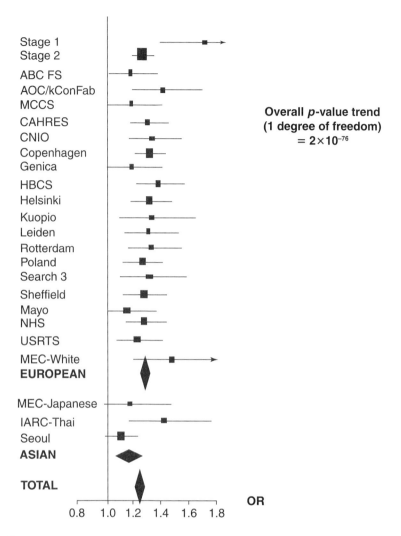

Figure 6
Consistent results across study centres for the top 'hit' (FGFR2) in stage 3 of the genome-wide association study.

What can we infer about the remaining 95% of genes? The study had sufficient power (93%) to identify the top hit, so it seems unlikely that there are many common variants of this size of effect. Conversely, the study had very poor power to detect the fourth and fifth hits (~1–3%), which implies that there could be hundreds more with similar or smaller effects – for example, the *CASP8* SNP did not reach the required statistical significance in stage I. The contribution of rare events and variants with a frequency of 1–10% is still uncertain, as is how many alleles it will be possible to identify.

Practical implications

Strong genes such as *BRCA1* and *BRCA2*, which have a relative risk of around 20, are very rare, so the population attributable fraction – the proportion of breast cancer removed if the effect of that variant is removed – is very small (about 2%). Conversely, although the top hit in the genome-wide study is much weaker and has a relative risk of only about 1.3 in heterozygotes, it is common and thus has a population attributable fraction of 16–18%. If it were possible to find a method of neutralizing the effect of that variant in women with one or two copies of the variant allele, the overall incidence of breast cancer could in principle be reduced by 16–18%, although the potential extent of collateral damage is unknown. As mentioned earlier, about 50% of the genetic variation probably needs to be identified to allow clinically useful prediction of an individual's risk, but only 5% has thus far been identified. Developments over the next few years will provide an indication of whether the 50% goal is achievable, but it will depend on the genetic architecture of the predisposition.

In terms of clinical interventions, it may be possible to identify high-risk groups and thus target interventions. In this case, the targeted preventive intervention may be mechanism-specific or generic. If woman are in high-risk groups because of the combined effect of 10–50 genes, however, it will still be necessary to use generic interventions, because any individual mechanism is likely to be only a small contributor to the reason the woman is at high risk. Another approach might be to target the attributable risk of a common allele across the population more generally. This is likely to be mechanism-based and analogous to the situation with cholesterol or blood pressure.

References

1. Antoniou A, Pharoah PDP, Narod S et al. Average risks of breast and ovarian cancer associated with *BRCA1* or *BRCA2* mutations detected in case series unselected for family history: a combined analysis of 22 studies. *Am J Hum Genet* 2003; **72**: 1117–21.
2. Ponder BAJ, Antoniou A, Dunning A et al. Polygenic inherited predisposition to breast cancer. *Cold Spring Harb Symp Quant Biol* 2005; **70**: 35–41.
3. Easton DF. How many more breast cancer predisposition genes are there? *Breast Cancer Res* 1999; **1**: 14–17.
4. Pharoah PDP, Antoniou A, Bobrow M et al. Polygenic susceptibility to breast cancer and implications for prevention. *Nat Genet* 2002; **31**: 33–6.
5. Pharoah PDP, Dunning AM, Ponder BAJ, Easton DP. Association studies for finding cancer-susceptibility genetic variants. *Nat Rev Cancer* 2004; **4**: 850–60.
6. Wang WYS, Barratt BJ, Clayton DG, Todd JA. Genome-wide association studies: theoretical and practical concerns. *Nat Rev Genet* 2005; **6**: 109–18.
7. Hinds DA, Sture LL, Nilsen GB et al. Whole genome patterns of common DNA variation in three human populations. *Science* 2005; **307**: 1072–9.
8. Easton DF, 102 others and Ponder BAJ. Genome-wide association study identifies novel breast cancer susceptibility loci. *Nature* 2007; **447**: 1087–93.

Lessons about cancer from cluster analysis

PAUL ELLIOTT

Investigation of the occurrence of cancers in clusters can be either reactive or proactive. Reactive investigations are done in response to reports of an excess of disease or cancer in a particular area. Such reports usually result from someone linking the disease to a source of environmental pollution, and may be made in the local press, by the local public health doctor or by worried patients or their families. The first step in a reactive investigation is to determine whether or not there is a true excess of cancer in the area, as many such putative clusters do not stand up to detailed investigation. This is done with reference to the expected numbers of cancers (based on national or regional rates) in a defined population over a particular period. If an apparent excess is found, then usually it is not possible to ascertain from the reported data alone whether there might be a causative link to the suggested source. Possible links can be extremely difficult to unravel, as it is often unclear whether the association with the putative source was made post hoc, after the identification of high disease rates in the study area, thus invalidating formal statistical appraisal. It is therefore often necessary to consider whether or not there is an excess in other areas with similar sources of pollution or perhaps in a different time period to confirm persistency. The second type of investigation is proactive; this involves an a priori test of a hypothesis of excess disease risk around a source of pollution without prior knowledge of the rates of disease in the area. This type of approach is more embedded in standard hypothesis testing, and the statistics are more tractable.[1]

A number of different approaches can also be used to investigate the occurrence of disease in areas to detect possible clusters or clustering, i.e. the tendency for cases of the disease to occur non-randomly in the population. Disease mapping has been undertaken for many years at international, national and local scales. The idea is to identify patterns of disease and perhaps link them to putative environmental causes. Whereas investigation of a specific disease cluster that has come to the attention of the authorities may be undertaken in a particular area, as already noted, a more generalized approach to disease clustering looks at the pattern of disease across areas much more broadly – in other words, investigating whether a cancer occurs generally in a clustered process. This may give clues as to aetiology; for example, Hodgkin lymphoma seems to occur in a clustered fashion, suggesting a possible infectious aetiology. This chapter focuses on disease mapping, particularly across small areas, and cluster investigation, and will also consider whether surveillance of large databases should be undertaken to try and identify possible clusters of disease.

Disease mapping

In Figure 1, the incidence of liver cancer in men around the world shows wide-scale geographical variability, with high rates in China, Eastern Asia and parts of Africa and lower rates in the developed world.[2] This largely mirrors the incidence of infection with hepatitis B and

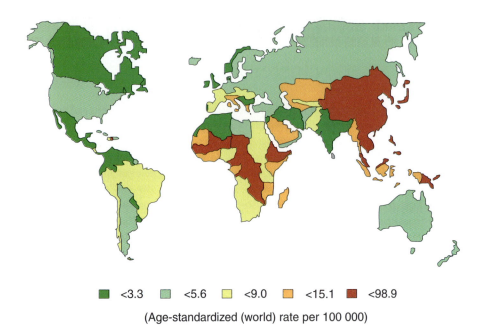

<3.3   <5.6   <9.0   <15.1   <98.9

(Age-standardized (world) rate per 100 000)

Figure 1
Disease surveillance at the international level: age-standardized (world) rate of liver cancer in men per 100 000.[2]

hepatitis C and thus reflects the geographical distribution of the major underlying cause. At the national level, Figure 2 shows the relative incidence of malignant melanoma of skin in women in England and Wales at district level.[3] Some of the highest rates are found in the southwest of England, where people are exposed to the largest amounts of sunshine. The incidence of malignant melanoma thus may also reflect a causative geographical association with an underlying environmental exposure, in this case ultraviolet radiation.

Patterns become more complex at the local (small-area) scale. Figure 3(a) shows a disease map for leukaemia in the West Midlands over a 13-year period that suggests a 2–3-fold variation in incidence rates and indicates some areas with apparently high risks of leukaemia.[4] Conceivably, such rates might be linked by the media or the public to a factory or polluting chimney in the area; that is, there could be an apparent contextual overlay of disease rates and putative cause. The problem at the local scale, however, is that the map is dominated by random variation. When the geographical variation is smoothed out to remove the random component, the disease map becomes flat (Figure 3(b)). Some residual variability is still apparent, because leukaemia is not completely randomly distributed, but the apparent clustering of high rates in certain areas is no longer seen. Areas with an apparently high incidence in the unsmoothed map may have small populations: for example, wards in the centre of Birmingham will have bigger populations than wards in the outskirts of the city. Reports of high incidences of leukaemia in the periphery of major towns may reflect such artefacts. There are, therefore, major problems of interpretation of disease maps at the local level, with so-called clusters in

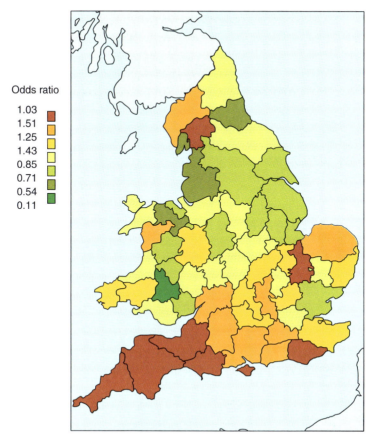

Figure 2
Disease surveillance at the national level: malignant melanoma of the skin in women in England and Wales, 1965–83.[3]

small areas often resulting from small numbers, small denominators and a lot of random variability.[1] For the commoner cancers, however, such as lung cancer, real variability in disease rates may be apparent at a local scale, reflecting variations in underlying causative lifestyle factors such as smoking.

Figure 4 shows the relative incidence of lung cancer according to the Carstairs index (an indicator of deprivation based on census statistics at a small-area level, in which the higher the Carstairs score the more deprived is the area).[5] At the level of census wards, a broad correlation is seen between the risk of lung cancer and the Carstairs index; a 2–3-fold variation in risk is noted purely on the basis of the census statistics used to calculate the Carstairs index (unemployment, overcrowding, social class and car ownership). At the local level, therefore, a large variability in cancer rates may potentially reflect lifestyle habits associated with deprivation (e.g. smoking) rather than the effects of environmental pollution.

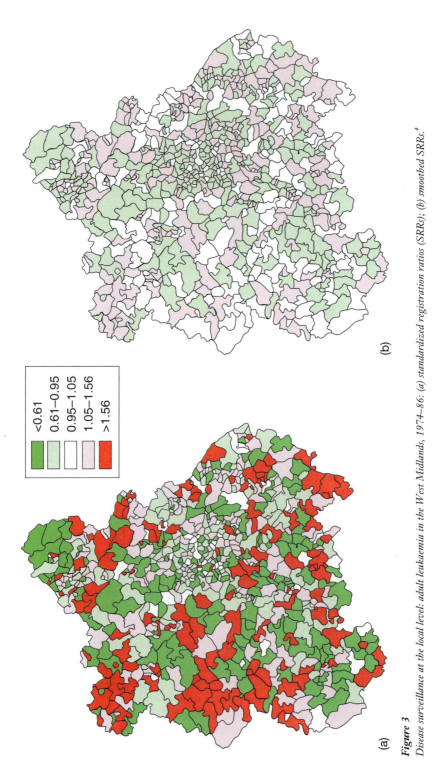

	<0.61
	0.61–0.95
	0.95–1.05
	1.05–1.56
	>1.56

(a)

(b)

Figure 3
Disease surveillance at the local level: adult leukaemia in the West Midlands, 1974–86: (a) standardized registration ratios (SRRs); (b) smoothed SRRs.[4]

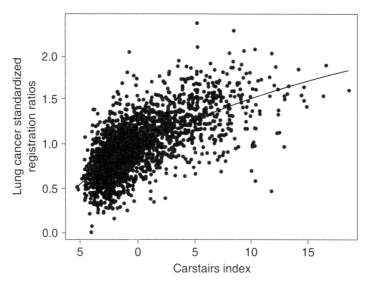

Figure 4
Standardized registration ratios relating incidence of lung cancer to score on the Carstairs index in the Thames region of England.[5]

Cluster investigations

In May 1996, national newspapers described 'parents' fears in poison town' after 'three children in the same classroom contract[ed] leukaemia' and reported a 'leukaemia cluster at school in town hit by pollution'. These media reports reflected widespread local concern about potential clusters of cancer and other diseases as a result of the deposition of aluminium sulphate into the water supply in Camelford, North Cornwall several years previously. One problem with reports such as these is that there is often no hypothesis – they simply reflect post hoc reports where people have noticed a high incidence of cancer or another disease in the area. Because the affected areas are small, there is a lot of random variability. As areas with low rates of cancer or disease are never reported, this results in a bias towards reporting apparently high incidences that may in fact reflect random variability – or statistical artefacts. Once a putative cluster is observed, a suspect source of pollution will often soon be 'identified' and damned by association, which, as already noted, invalidates formal statistical testing. In addition, reports from small areas are often dominated by data errors or anomalies: the cancers or diseases in the cluster may be duplicate cases, they may be cases of different cancers that would not be expected to share a common aetiology or there may be problems with the denominator that will result in incorrect expected rates of disease. Finally, another common feature of such investigations is so-called boundary shrinkage – three cases may occur in a classroom, but that classroom is in a school, which is in a district, which is in a town ... and the smaller the boundary drawn around the cases, the smaller is the denominator and the higher the apparent risk.[6]

Concerning the investigation of individual clusters, Alexander and Cuzick[7] asserted that reports 'can be justified from a scientific point of view only if [this] leads to identification of an aetiological factor which is a substantial cause of the total burden of the disease [or] an overwhelming cause of the disease in a particular area.' In other words, the risk has to be extremely high for cluster investigations to bear fruit – and, unfortunately, most of them do not.

A cluster in High Wycombe, Berkshire, provides an example where there was a very high risk of disease due to a specific cause.[8] In this case, it was an occupational cause – working in the furniture industry in the High Wycombe area. The very high risk of adenocarcinoma of the nasal sinuses was detected not by any systematic trawling through the data but by an alert clinician. Indeed, a doctor suddenly encountering more than the usual number of patients with a very rare disease is often the manner in which clusters come to attention.

Probably the most well-known cluster is the leukaemia cluster around the Windscale nuclear power plant at Sellafield. It was identified in 1983, not by public health authorities or a systematic review of the local health statistics, but by a team who set out to make a television documentary about the workforce but ended up making a documentary about children and young people in the area who were developing high rates of leukaemia and non-Hodgkin lymphoma. Their findings led to a government inquiry headed by Sir Douglas Black, which confirmed an excess of leukaemia and lymphoma in young people in the area.[9] Among a number of recommendations, the Black Inquiry noted that there was no ready means of looking at the cancer statistics in the area; it was a major task to obtain data for the local area and make estimates of the local occurrence of disease. The enquiry recommended that 'encouragement should be given to an organization … to co-ordinate centrally the monitoring of small area statistics around major installations producing discharges that might present a carcinogenic or mutagenic hazard to the public. In this way, early warning of any untoward health effect could be obtained.' Thus the inquiry team noted the need to look not just at nuclear installations but at other installations that might be producing carcinogenic hazards. The inquiry also recommended an early warning system involving surveillance of health statistics; however, this is not as straightforward as it might seem, as discussed later in this chapter.

As a result of the Black Inquiry recommendation, the UK Small Area Health Statistics Unit (SAHSU) was established, initially at the London School of Hygiene and Tropical Medicine and latterly at Imperial College London,[10] with a number of aims:

- to develop and maintain a comprehensive database of health data, using the postcode that identifies a building or street to provide a very high-resolution geographical code
- to develop and maintain relevant databases of environmental exposures and social confounding factors at the small-area level (because disease occurrence is not random and reflects the lifestyle and deprivation of an area)
- to carry out substantive research studies on environment and health, including studies of socio-economic factors and health (again reflecting the fact that socio-economic factors are predominant for many of these diseases)
- to respond rapidly to ad hoc queries about unusual clusters of disease, particularly in the neighbourhood of industrial installations (this is a specific task to determine whether or not putative clusters are confirmed in the national statistics)

- to develop and maintain a rapid inquiry facility (that can look quickly at reports of disease excess in particular areas)
- to develop small-area statistical methods (after the Sellafield cluster, this was a new area of statistical endeavour)

The unit collects event data on births, deaths, cancers, hospital admissions and other health datasets such as congenital anomalies. These are tagged by postcode, which allows a map grid reference to be identified so that cases can be located to within about 100 m. Areas for analysis are then identified; these may reflect administrative boundaries such as wards or districts, the area within a specified distance from a possible source, or a plume around a source of pollution. Census data on the population are used to calculate risks and rates. The methods can be illustrated with the help of Figure 5, which in this case shows the electoral wards from which population data are drawn (enumeration districts or census output areas might also be used). The central point represents a putative source of pollution that is proposed to be causing disease in the area. The postcodes in which people live are identified by red crosses. Areas for analysis, in this case circular areas, are drawn up using a Geographical Information System. The underlying census areas are also used to identify other characteristics of places and people who live in them. In this case, the wards are coloured to denote whether they are urban (brown) or rural (green), but equally they could denote deprivation scores or other areal characteristics.

This approach was used to investigate reports of a putative cluster made by a GP who claimed there was an excess of leukaemia in his practice very close to the television and radio transmitter at Sutton Coldfield near Birmingham. The rates of leukaemia and other cancers near the Sutton Coldfield transmitter were identified from the national database held within SAHSU. A basic model based on distance was used to look at decline in risk of leukaemia with distance from the transmitter.[11] One case occurred within 500 m when only 0.1 case was expected, another 5 cases occurred within 1 km when 2.7 would be expected and 17 occurred within 1–2 km when 10 would be expected: within 2 km, therefore, an 80% excess of leukaemia was found between 1974 and 1986 in comparison with age-, sex- and regionally adjusted national rates. The initial investigation thus confirmed an apparent excess of leukaemia near the transmitter. The next question, of course, was whether this excess was related to the transmitter. On the basis of the initial findings, the study was extended to all other television and radio transmitters in the UK to independently test the hypothesis that an excess of leukaemia cases occurs near radio and television transmitters. The magnitude and pattern of leukaemia risk around the other transmitters did not reflect that around Sutton Coldfield, so the conclusion was that the excess near Sutton Coldfield was unlikely to be related to its proximity to the transmitter.[12]

In another example, we are using an a priori approach to determine whether there is a high incidence of childhood cancer near mobile phone base stations and, if so, whether this might be related to transmissions from the base stations. This is a very different scenario from a post hoc cluster investigation in which someone has suggested an excess of childhood cancer in a particular area and then noted a base station nearby: in this study, we have no prior knowledge of the health statistics around any of the base stations. The study is investigating the incidence of leukaemia, non-Hodgkin lymphoma and all childhood cancers in children aged 0–4 years over a 3-year period in Great Britain. We have obtained data on cases from the national cancer register with birth date- and sex-matched controls selected from the national

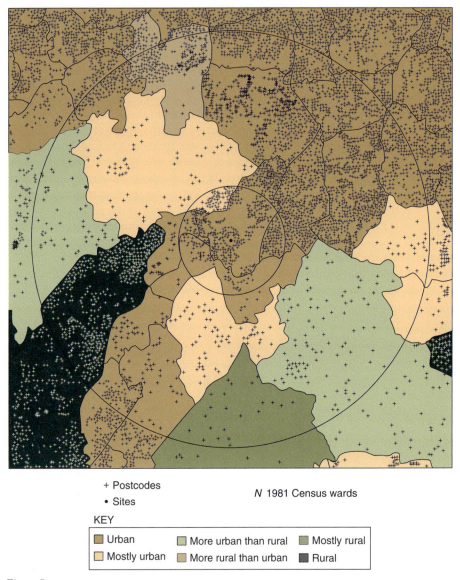

+ Postcodes
• Sites

N 1981 Census wards

KEY

⬛ Urban	🟩 More urban than rural	🟩 Mostly rural
⬜ Mostly urban	🟫 More rural than urban	⬛ Rural

Figure 5
Link between postcodes (health events) and underlying geography around a point source.

birth register. As exposure from a base station falls off very quickly with distance, the postcode system does not provide high enough geographical resolution, so we are using individual addresses. We are considering distance from nearest base station as a basic metric, total power output from nearby base stations, as well as modelling power density at each child's address and calibrating the model via a number of field surveys.

Issues with cluster detection

As noted above, the Black Inquiry into the leukaemia cluster at Sellafield called for an 'early warning' system based on analysis of the national statistics. However, surveillance of the large databases that cover all cancer registrations, mortality and hospital admissions for the UK is problematic for a number of reasons. These include the variable quality of data and the difficulty in differentiating between false- and true-positive findings when identifying putative clusters of disease. The low excess relative risk of chronic diseases such as cancer that has been associated with environmental pollution also makes clusters very difficult to detect reliably. Multiple testing is a major problem, as it is necessary to look at different ages, both sexes, and the full range of diseases in different areas and over different time periods. Potential confounding because of differences in lifestyle and levels of deprivation between areas, as mentioned earlier, is another important consideration. This is further complicated by the need to define the sensitivity and specificity of the surveillance system, which is, essentially, a public health screening test. All in all, routine surveillance of the national health statistics has not so far been carried out for the above reasons.

Summary

Disease mapping may indicate areas of high risk of disease and suggest clues as to aetiology. Rates identified at the small-area scale may be unstable because of small numbers. Patterns of disease may be dominated by variations in socio-economic and lifestyle factors, such as smoking. Most cluster investigations are unlikely to reveal new causes of disease unless the risks are very high. Surveillance of the routine statistics to detect disease clusters is not currently carried out because of concerns about both false-positive and false-negative findings.

References

1. Elliott P, Wartenberg D. Spatial epidemiology: current approaches and future challenges. *Environ Health Perspect* 2004; **112**: 998–1006.
2. Parkin DM. International variation. *Oncogene* 2004; **23**: 6329–40.
3. Swerdlow A, dos Santos Silva I. *Atlas of Cancer Incidence in England and Wales 1968–85*. Oxford: Oxford University Press, 1993.
4. Eaton N, Shaddick G, Dolk H, Elliott P. Small-area study of the incidence of neoplasms of the brain and cerebral nervous system in the West Midlands region, 1974–86. *Br J Cancer* 1997; **75**: 1080–3.
5. Carstairs V. Socio-economic factors at area level and their relationship with health. In: Elliott P, Wakefield J, Best N, Briggs D, eds. *Spatial Epidemiology: Methods and Applications*. Oxford: Oxford University Press, 2000: 51–67.
6. Olsen SF, Martuzzi M, Elliott P. Cluster analysis and disease mapping – why, when, and how? A step by step guide. *BMJ* 1996; **313**: 863–6.
7. Alexander FE, Cuzick J. Methods for the assessment of disease clusters. In: Elliott P, Cuzick J, English D, Stern R, eds. *Geographical and Environmental Epidemiology: Methods for Small-Area Studies*. Oxford: Oxford University Press, 1992.
8. Acheson ED, Cowdell RH, Hadfield E, Macbeth RG. Nasal cancer in woodworkers in the furniture industry. *BMJ* 1968; **2**(5605): 587–96.
9. Black D. *Investigation of the Possible Increased Incidence of Cancer in West Cumbria. Report of the Independent Advisory Group*. London: HMSO, 1984.
10. Elliott P, Westlake AJ, Hills M et al. The Small Area Health Statistics Unit: a national facility for investigating health around point sources of environmental pollution in the United Kingdom. *J Epidemiol Community Health* 1992; **46**: 345–9.

11. Dolk H, Shaddick G, Walls P et al. Cancer incidence near radio and television transmitters in Great Britain. I. Sutton Coldfield transmitter. *Am J Epidemiol* 1997; **145**: 1–9.
12. Dolk H, Elliott P, Shaddick G et al. Cancer incidence near high power radio and TV transmitters in Great Britain: II. All transmitter sites. *Am J Epidemiol* 1997; **145**: 10–17.

Section Two: Environmental Culprits

The role of nutrition in cancer aetiology and prevention

ELIO RIBOLI

Interest in the possible relation between nutrition and cancer has grown substantially over the past two decades. One reason for this is the perception in the 1960s and 1970s that the incidence of some cancers, particularly those of the colon, breast and prostate, was increasing in the populations of Western Europe and North America with no clear link to any chemical or physical carcinogens. As these changes in incidence could not be accommodated in the traditional chemical view of carcinogenesis, attention shifted towards metabolic and lifestyle factors, including diet.

The so-called Western lifestyle has been characterized by a substantial increase in the energy density of the diet over the past few decades. This mainly consists of an increase in the consumption of fat, refined carbohydrates (sugar) and animal protein in parallel with a progressive reduction in physical activity. Until recently, people in rural China, for example, were estimated to expend about 4000–5000 kilocalories per day in their normal activities, so that, although they ate a large number of calories, they would be lean. Most relatively active people in the Western world expend about 2500–3000 kilocalories per day, but although they eat less than the rural Chinese people described above, they move even less than is needed to burn off the calories consumed, and this underlies the Western epidemic of obesity. Smoking and drinking also contribute, with variable patterns over time in different countries. The consequences are very complex and difficult to disentangle, but adult body height has increased greatly and major changes have occurred in some key physiological metabolic characteristics, such as earlier menarche. In addition, there is an increased prevalence of obesity, cardiovascular risk factors and conditions, diabetes, and hypertension.

With this in mind, more than 15 years ago, the International Agency for Research on Cancer (IARC) decided to improve knowledge about diet and cancer by taking advantage of large variations in the incidence of cancer and in the diets and lifestyles of European populations. For example, gastric cancer is more frequent in the south of Europe than in the north, but prostate cancer is more frequent in the north than in the south. As a result, the European Prospective Investigation into Cancer and Nutrition (EPIC) was set up in 1993 and has now collected and stored personal data and blood from more than 400 000 participants.

Prospective core studies such as this are lifetime engagements, starting with the collection of baseline data, continuing with follow-up of cancer diagnosis, vital status, causes of death and changes and lifestyles, and concluding with aetiological studies. All participants in the EPIC study have been approached 1–3 times to measure changes in lifestyle, and this in-built design allows us to identify when patients, for example, give up smoking, modify their lifestyle or become menopausal in the case of women.

This chapter will now look at the findings of the EPIC study in relation to breast cancer and colorectal cancer.

Colorectal cancer

One of the earliest hypotheses in relation to diet and colorectal cancer was the Burke hypothesis on fibres, which was put forward after populations with a very high intake of plant food were observed to have a much lower risk of colorectal cancer. The hypothesis gained momentum as a result of case–control studies conducted in the 1970s and 1980s, at which point the claim that fibre reduced the risk of colorectal cancer was accepted in the USA. A few years ago, however, a series of studies from North America found no association between fibre and colorectal cancer, and this resulted in the Kellogg Company removing from their cereal boxes the claim that fibre reduces the risk of colorectal cancer.

In 2003, the EPIC researchers, having been able to investigate a very broad range of exposures to dietary fibre (from <15 to >35 g/day), showed an almost linear decrease in the incidence of colorectal cancer with increasing consumption of fibre in the form of cereals, fruit, vegetables and legumes (Figure 1). They also twice measured consumption of fibre in about 40 000 participants to adjust for some imprecision in the measurement of diet; this is the only study to have used this calibration approach. The results showed that if the 50% of the population that consumes <25 g of fibre/day consumed >25 g/day like the other 50% of the population, the incidence of colorectal cancer would be reduced by 30–40%. These findings were strengthened from a biological point of view by the simultaneous publication of similar results from a study on colorectal adenoma in the USA,[2] which indicated that fibre most likely acts

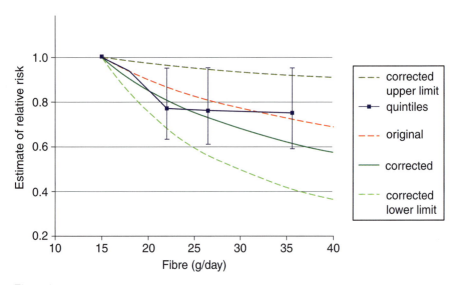

Figure 1
Colorectal cancer and dietary fibre. Statistical model adjusted for energy, height, weight, physical activity, alcohol and tobacco. Reproduced with permission from Bingham et al.[1]

on the entire pathogenetic process – from the normal mucosa down to the development of carcinogenesis. A group from Harvard led by Walter Willett was concerned about possible confounding on the basis that people who eat more fibre also eat more vegetables and therefore consume more folate, but a reanalysis of data showed that these are independent effects.[3]

Results from the EPIC study that have potential implications for prevention are those on 'animal food'.[4] The key result is confirmation of previous reports that consumption of red meat (beef, lamb and pork) and processed meat is associated with a significant 20–40% increase in the risk of colorectal cancer, while consumption of fish is associated with a 30–40% decrease in risk (Figure 2). Although the relative risks are modest compared, for example, with the risk of smoking, when the relative risks are combined, even a relatively low level of intake at the population level produces a non-negligible risk. Figure 3 illustrates the combined effects of consumption of red meat and fibre and consumption of fish and fibre, and shows that the risk increases with increasing level of red meat intake and decreasing level of fibre intake. Similar results are seen with consumption of fibre and fish. This strongly suggests that the two factors act independently from a statistical point of view, in the sense that low levels of fish consumption of are associated with an increased risk and low levels of fibre consumption are associated with an increased risk, for whichever level of the other variable.

Why would red meat but not poultry or fish be associated with an increased risk of colon cancer? The answer may have been provided by Bingham's experiments on volunteers, which showed that endogenous production of faecal N-nitroso compounds increased when people switched from a diet low in red meat to a diet high in red meat, and then decreased again when they switched to a vegetarian diet (Figure 4).[5] This pattern was replicated when people switched from a diet low in red meat to a diet high in red meat and then to a diet high in white

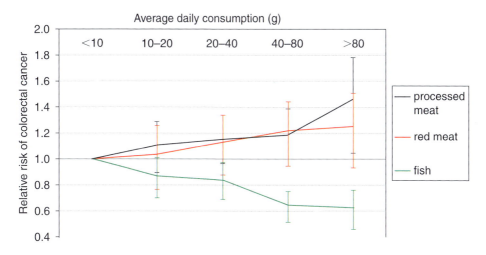

Figure 2
Colorectal cancer, fish and red and processed meats. Statistical model adjusted for energy, height, weight, physical activity, fibre, alcohol and tobacco. Reproduced with permission from Norat et al.[4]

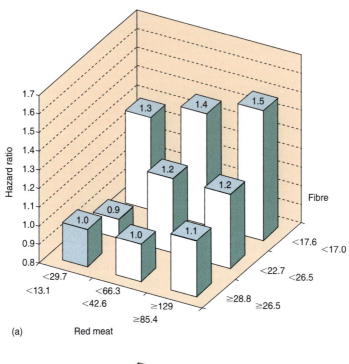

(a)

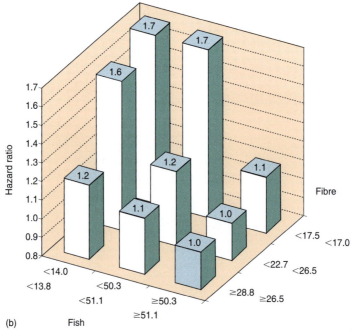

(b)

Figure 3

Combined effects of consumption of red meat and fibre (a) and fish and fibre (b). Reproduced with permission from Norat et al.[4]

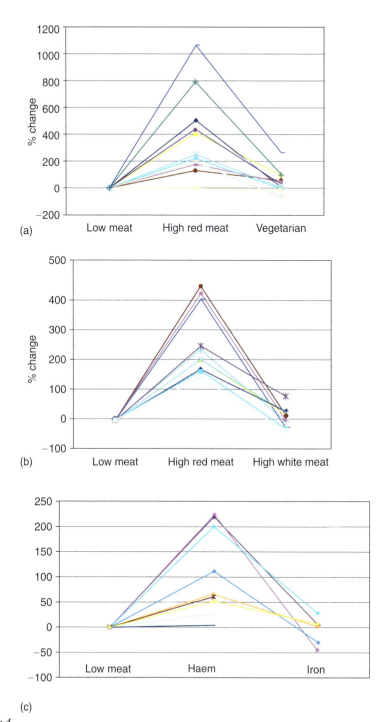

(a)

(b)

(c)

Figure 4

Changes in levels of faecal N-nitroso compounds according to dietary intake of meat, haem and iron. Reproduced with permission from Cross et al.[5]

meat. The researchers then switched volunteers from a diet low in meat to a diet containing iron in the form of haem (the substance that makes red meat red) and then to a diet containing iron in the form found in vitamin supplements – and replicated the same pattern. Iron in the form of haem thus catalyses the endogenous formation of N-nitroso compounds and might contribute towards the difference between red and white meat.

The other major area of development in the past decade has been the accumulation of overwhelming evidence that physical activity, height and weight are associated with colorectal cancer. Results from the EPIC study show an almost linear relation between the incidence of colorectal cancer and height after adjustment for other factors (Table 1), which suggests that some event early in life, perhaps before the age of 18–20 years, leaves an imprint that results in an increased risk of colorectal cancer. The effect is seen in both sexes, but is stronger in women; it is also replicated with respect to breast cancer. This is not a trivial finding when the major increase in height observed over the past 150 years, which represents a major change in human physiology, is taken into account. For example, the average height of men entering military service in the Netherlands has increased by 20 cm just through changes in lifestyle and nutrition, and this could account for a large proportion of the observed increase in the incidence of colorectal cancer.

Results from the EPIC study in terms of body mass index (BMI), which is a marker of obesity, confirmed the findings of many other studies in men, namely a linear increase in the incidence of colorectal cancer (Table 2). No such association was seen in women. The researchers therefore investigated abdominal obesity in women (men were not included, as >90% of men have abdominal obesity) and found a significant association with a risk of colorectal cancer. Interestingly, women who were not taking hormone replacement therapy (HRT) did not show an increase in cancer. For the first time for colorectal cancer, these results replicated an

Table 1 Colorectal cancer and height in men and women. Reproduced with permission from Pischon et al[6]

Height (cm)	Odds ratio	
	Crude	Adjusted
Men		
<168.0	1 (referent)	1 (referent)
168.0–172.4	1.09 (0.79–1.50)	1.10 (0.80–1.52)
172.5–176.1	1.14 (0.82 –1.57)	1.16 (0.84–1.60)
176.2–180.4	1.14 (0.82–1.57)	1.29 (0.93–1.79)
≥180.5	1.14 (0.82–1.57)	1.40 (0.99–1.98)
p-trend	0.06	0.04
Women		
<156.0	1 (referent)	1 (referent)
156.0–172.4	1.34 (0.99–1.80)	1.33 (0.99–1.80)
160.5–176.1	1.72 (1.29–2.30)	1.71 (1.28–2.28)
163.2–180.4	1.68 (1.25–2.27)	1.66 (1.23–2.24)
≥167.5	1.82 (1.33–2.50)	1.79 (1.30–2.46)
p-trend	0.001	0.001

Table 2   *Colorectal cancer and body mass index (BMI) in men and women. Reproduced with permission from Pischon et al[6]*

BMI (kg/m^2)	Odds ratio	
	Crude	Adjusted
Men		
<23.6	1 (referent)	1 (referent)
23.6–25.3	1.20 (0.86–1.66)	1.18 (0.85–1.63)
25.4–27.0	1.03 (0.74–1.45)	1.00 (0.71–1.41)
27.1–29.3	1.24 (0.89–1.72)	1.19 (0.85–1.66)
≥29.4	1.64 (1.19– 2.25)	1.55 (1.12–2.15)
p-trend	0.002	0.006
Women		
<21.7	1 (referent)	1 (referent)
21.7–23.5	1.09 (0.79–1.50)	1.09 (0.79–1.50)
23.6–25.7	1.14 (0.82 –1.57)	1.14 (0.82–1.57)
25.8–28.8	1.14 (0.82–1.57)	1.14 (0.82–1.57)
≥28.9	1.14 (0.82–1.57)	1.14 (0.82–1.57)
p-trend	0.46	0.40

effect already reported for breast cancer – the use of HRT masks the effect of obesity. This may explain why a review found that all case–control studies reported a stronger association in men than in women.[7]

The variable most likely to impact on the risk of colorectal cancer thus seems to be abdominal obesity – but why is this the case? In 2000, Kaaks et al[8] postulated that the mechanism might actually be insulin resistance, which is strongly associated with abdominal obesity, and that high levels of insulin could increase the risk of colorectal cancer and possibly breast cancer. Indeed, the consequent prospective study in 15 000 women in New York found that C-peptide, which is a relatively good marker of high levels of insulin production, had a linear association with an increased risk of colorectal cancer, with a relative risk of 3. This study was reproduced in the much larger EPIC population; although the relative risk decreased to 1.7, which is probably more realistic, it still shows a clear effect of insulin resistance adjusted for BMI.[9]

The key results of the EPIC study to date have shown that a number of factors, including dietary factors, metabolic factors, alcohol and tobacco (probably in the early stages), are associated with an increased risk of colorectal cancer. This will allow a model of an environment for intervention to be developed.

Breast cancer

Although modifiable risk factors, such as diet, have been identified for colorectal cancer, the situation is very different for breast cancer. Investigations into the effect of diet have not produced any strong associations, and a recent report noted that total or specific vegetable and fruit intake is not associated with a risk of breast cancer.[9]

Research over the past 20 years has identified a number of metabolic factors that are strongly associated with breast cancer. The age of menarche has been decreasing in European countries over the past 150 years: from 17 years to an average of just 11 years 8 months in the USA.[10] This is extremely important, as many studies have shown that early menarche is associated with an increased risk of breast cancer later in life. In China, for example, there is a 40% reduction in the risk of breast cancer in women who had late menarche.[11] Height is also associated with an increased risk, and, as mentioned earlier, this is a marker of an event in terms of diet, protein intake or insulin production before the age of 20 years. Unfortunately, however, both of these unmodifiable factors are difficult to use to prevent breast cancer developing after the age of 50 years.

A linear increase is seen for weight gain between the ages of 20 and 60 years and the risk of breast cancer. In premenopausal women, there is no association with breast cancer and possibly even a very weak reduction in risk, while there is a 30–40% increased risk in postmenopausal women. It is important to separate postmenopausal women who do and do not take HRT, however, because such treatment overwhelmingly masks the effect of weight gain and BMI at a given age. The biological basis for this, in fact, is very strong. Data from 1192 postmenopausal women in the EPIC study illustrate that as BMI increases, levels of free testosterone and estrone in the blood increase and levels of sex hormone-binding globulin (SHBG), which is a major factor in the risk of breast cancer, decrease. SHBG is produced by the liver, binds inactive forms of hormones and is regulated by insulin, so the higher the levels of insulin in the blood, the lower the levels of SHBG and the higher the levels of free estradiol. This was shown quite clearly by the results of the EPIC study regarding steroid hormones – with the risk of breast cancer increasing with increasing levels of testosterone, estrone, androstenedione, free testosterone and free estradiol, and decreasing with increasing levels of SHBG (Figure 5).

In premenopausal women, however, a very different pattern is seen, with an increased risk of breast cancer being associated with high levels of testosterone, androstenedione and all androgens, but not with SHBG or the estrogens.[13] To further complicate matters, the EPIC researchers have recently reported that insulin resistance is associated with a decreased risk of breast cancer before menopause.

In conclusion, the reality behind the metabolic factors that influence the risk of breast cancer is much more complex than previously thought, with factors at work before the menopause not being important after the menopause.

Table 3 *Colorectal cancer and waist circumference in women. Reproduced with permission from Pischon et al*[6]

Waist circumference (cm)	Women who take HRT	Women who do not take HRT
<70.2	1 (referent)	1 (referent)
70.2–75.8	1.30 (0.80–2.11)	1.07 (0.55–2.06)
75.9–80.9	1.35 (0.85–2.14)	0.79 (0.39–1.57)
81.0–88.9	1.39 (0.88–2.19)	0.90 (0.44–1.83)
≥89.0	1.68 (1.06–2.64)	0.76 (0.32–1.80)
p-trend	0.02	0.46

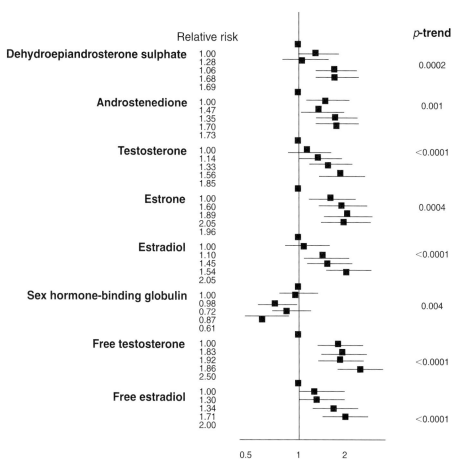

Figure 5
Postmenopausal serum sex steroids and the risk of breast cancer. Reproduced with permission from Kaaks et al.[12]

References

1.   Bingham SA, Day NE, Luben R et al. Dietary fibre in food an d protection against colorectal cancer in the European Prospective Investigation into Cancer and Nutrition (EPIC): an observational study. *Lancet* 2003; **361**: 1496–501.

2.   Peter U, Sinha R, Chatterjee N et al. Dietary fibre and colorectal adenoma in a colorectal cancer early detection programme. *Lancet* 2003; **361**: 1491–5.

3.   Bingham SA, Norat T, Moskal A et al. Is the association with fiber from foods in colorectal cancer confounded by folate intake? *Cancer Epidemiol Biomarkers Prev* 2005; **14**: 1552–6.

4.   Norat T, Bingham S, Ferrari P et al. Meat, fish, and colorectal cancer risk: the European Prospective Investigation into Cancer and Nutrition. *J Natl Cancer Inst* 2005; **97**: 906–16.

5.   Cross AJ, Pollock JR, Bingham SA. Red meat and colorectal cancer risk: the effect of dietary iron and haem on endogenous *N*-nitrosation. *IARC Sci Publ* 2002; **156**: 205–6.

6.   Pischon T, Lahmann PH, Boeing H et al. Body size and risk of colon and rectal cancer in the European Prospective Investigation Into Cancer and Nutrition (EPIC). *J Natl Cancer Inst* 2006; **98**: 920–31.

7. Lund Nilsen TI, Vatten LJ. Colorectal cancer associated with BMI, physical activity, diabetes, and blood glucose. *IARC Sci Publ* 2002; **156**: 257–8.

8. Kaaks R, Toniolo P, Akhmedkhanov A et al. Serum C-peptide, insulin-like growth factor (IGF)-I, IGF-binding proteins, and colorectal cancer risk in women. *J Natl Cancer Inst* 2000; **92**: 1592–600.

9. van Gils CH, Peeters PH, Bueno-de-Mesquita HB et al. Consumption of vegetables and fruits and risk of breast cancer. *JAMA* 2005; **293**: 183–93.

10. Tanner JM. Trend towards earlier menarche in London, Oslo, Copenhagen, the Netherlands and Hungary. *Nature* 1973; **243**: 95–6.

11. Gao YT, Shu XO, Dai Q et al. Association of menstrual and reproductive factors with breast cancer risk: results from the Shanghai Breast Cancer Study. *Int J Cancer* 2000; **87**: 295–300.

12. Kaaks R, Rinaldi S, Key TJ et al. Postmenopausal serum androgens, oestrogens and breast cancer risk: the European prospective investigation into cancer and nutrition. *Endocr Relat Cancer* 2005; **12**: 1071–82.

13. Kaaks R, Berrino F, Key T et al. Serum sex steroids in premenopausal women and breast cancer risk within the European Prospective Investigation into Cancer and Nutrition (EPIC). *J Natl Cancer Inst* 2005; **97**: 755–65.

Smoking

Summarized from a presentation given by RICHARD PETO

Although this chapter reviews existing knowledge on smoking that is available on the website *Deaths from Smoking*,[1] it is included because it is not possible to discuss prevention of cancer without considering smoking, which accounts for such a large proportion of all cancer in the UK. Indeed, evidence from the UK is important, because people in the UK began smoking earlier than any other large population and continued at high levels for longer, which is the most effective way to ensure a smoking-related death.

Men born in the first few decades of the 20th century in the UK became the first large population in the world to smoke substantial numbers of cigarettes, and a fair number continue to do so. This population is important, therefore, because when a large increase in smoking in young people occurs, it is not until they reach old age that the full hazards become apparent. Indeed, studies of British men born in the first few decades of the 20th century are only now providing the first real glimpses of the dreadful consequences of this 'bad habit'. This delay in effects applies equally to women, although the hazards in women still cannot be fully studied: smoking in women was initially not 'respectable', and because regular smoking in young women did not start until the late 1950s and early 1960s, it is only when this cohort reaches old age that the full effects will be revealed.

The risks of smoking

The risks of smoking are enormous. Half of all smokers die from cancerous, vascular or respiratory smoking-related causes, with a quarter of these dying in middle age (35–69 years) and thus an unnecessary loss of many years of healthy life. Sir Richard Doll's data from male doctors born in the first few decades of the 20th century in the UK show a 25% difference in the proportion of smokers and lifelong non-smokers still alive at the age of 70 years (Figure 1). Mortality is considerably higher among smokers even at older ages: of the 58% of smokers still alive at the age of 70, half will die in the next 10 years, whereas far fewer than half of the 81 non-smokers will die in that period.[2]

Stopping smoking works remarkably well, given how effective smoking is at killing (Figure 2a).[2] On average, for men born between 1900 and 1930, cigarette smokers lost about 10 years of life, but smoking cessation at the ages of 60, 50, 40 and 30 years gained about 3, 6, 9 or almost the full 10 years, respectively.[1] Indeed, the pattern of mortality in people who smoke but stop at the age of 40 years is much more like the pattern for lifelong non-smokers than that for continuing cigarette smokers.[1] Although stopping smoking at any age reduces mortality from lung cancer, the earlier smoking is stopped the better (Figure 2b).[3]

Unpublished results from the first large prospective study of smoking and death in a population of women that included lifelong smokers show the full hazards in middle age of persistent cigarette smoking for women (Beral V, unpublished data, 2007). These data come from the Million Women Study, which included British women born around 1940 who attended

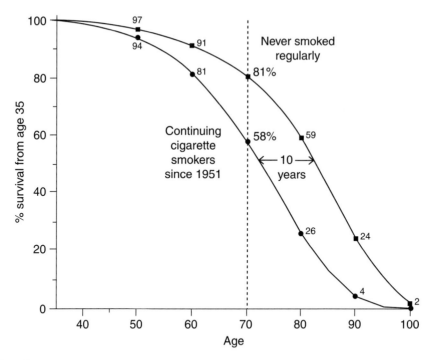

Figure 1

Survival in male doctors born between 1900 and 1930 who continued cigarette smoking since 1951 and those who never smoked, 1951–2001. Reproduced with permission from Doll et al.[2]

for breast cancer screening in the 1990s, many of whom have smoked seriously throughout adult life. For women who smoke around 15 cigarettes per day, overall mortality is around three times as great as for women who do not smoke; in other words, two-thirds of women who smoke 15 cigarettes a day and die in middle age would not have died were they non-smokers. The hazard is much higher for those who smoke 30 cigarettes a day, in whom 80% of deaths would not have occurred if the women did not smoke. In terms of vascular disease, women who smoke 15 cigarettes a day have a fourfold risk of dying of heart attack, a nearly fourfold risk of dying of stroke and about a fourfold risk of any sort of vascular-related death. The relative risks in women are more extreme than those observed in men of the same age range, although the absolute risks for woman are slightly smaller. The relative risk of lung cancer increases from zero in women who smoke no cigarettes per day to more than 50 in those who smoke 30 cigarettes a day. The data from this study also highlight the huge risks of smoking despite the fact that cigarette yields in the UK have been reduced in recent decades. This is important, because it confirms that modern low-tar cigarettes, which will have been smoked by most women since the 1970s and 1980s, are not safe and still result in high levels of mortality.

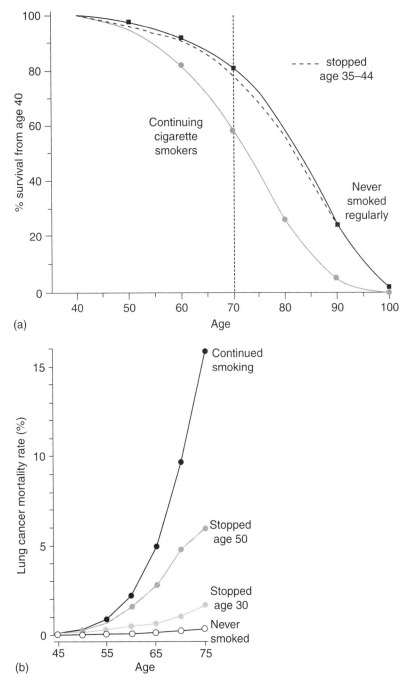

Figure 2
Effect of stopping smoking at about the age of 40 years on survival from age 40 years (a) and cumulative risk of and the effects of stopping smoking on lung cancer-related mortality (b). Reproduced with permission from Doll et al[2] (a) and Peto et al[3] (b).

33

Trends in mortality

In the USA, the first big increase in cigarette smoking occurred in the early 1900s, and this was followed by a general trend towards an increase in the number of cigarettes smoked daily until the last 20 years, when cigarette consumption per head halved. Increases were seen first in men and then later in women, and this is reflected in the patterns of cases of lung cancer (Figure 3a). In men, the huge increase in mortality from lung cancer is followed by the start of a decline in numbers; this contrasts with the trends in mortality of the other components of cancer mortality in the USA (Figure 3b). A similar but delayed and less pronounced pattern is seen in women (Figure 3c).

Data from studies that included around one million people and a few hundred thousand smokers in 1960 and 1980 confirmed smoking as the predominant cause of lung cancer, with mortality from lung cancer being unchanged in non-smokers but epidemic among smokers. The delay in development of lung cancer is key, however: the main increase in cigarette use in the first half of the 20th century in men and then women is followed by a main increase in death in the second half of the 20th century, again in men and then women. In 1950, only 12% of deaths in middle-aged Americans were caused by smoking, but it accounted for 33% of such deaths by 1990.

Age-standardized total cancer mortality had persistently increased in the USA since 1955 in men and was relatively constant in women. It had begun to decrease in the 1990s in both sexes, mainly because of a decrease in smoking-related deaths. Indeed, half of all cancer deaths in middle-aged American men – which means the loss of around 25 years of expected life per victim – were caused by smoking. Data therefore suggest that we are winning the war on cancer deaths caused by smoking. This is confirmed by lung cancer mortality figures in men and women aged 35–44 years, which halved between 1970 and 2000 (Figure 4). Over the next 20 years, the pattern seen in early middle-age will be repeated in later middle-age. As a result, data should eventually show much larger decreases in smoking-attributed cancer mortality in middle-age people in the USA than seen previously.

The effects of tobacco are even more dominant in the UK, which had the worst death rates from smoking in the world but now has the largest decrease as a result of the reduced prevalence of smoking (Figure 5). A fourfold decrease in lung cancer mortality has been seen in people aged 35–44 years in the UK since 1960. In 1970, 42 out of every 100 men in the UK would have died in middle-age, and 20 of those 42 deaths would have resulted from smoking; in 2000, 25 of every 100 men in Britain died in middle-age, and 6 of those 25 deaths would have resulted from smoking. The main reason for that decrease is that the probability of being killed by tobacco has decreased, in the population as a whole, from 20 to about 6.

In China, the major increase in cigarette smoking came around 40 years after the increase in the USA: American adults on average smoked one, four and 10 cigarettes per day in 1910, 1930 and 1950, while Chinese men on average smoked one, four and 10 cigarettes per day in 1952, 1972 and 1992, respectively. In the USA, 12% of deaths in middle-age were from smoking in 1950 and 33% in 1990; in Chinese men, 12% of deaths in 1990 were related to smoking. In China today, about two-thirds of young men smoke, and half of all smokers die

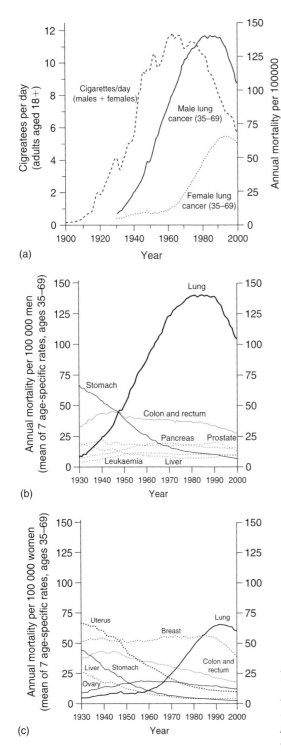

(a)

(b)

(c)

Figure 3

Trends in the USA: cigarette consumption and lung cancer mortality (a) and cancer mortality in men (b) and women (c). Reproduced with permission from Centers for Disease Control and Prevention.[4]

35

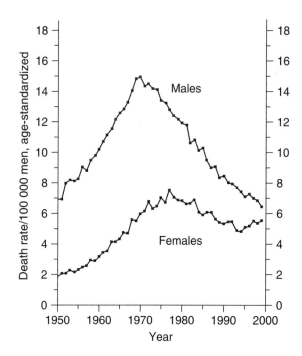

Figure 4

Lung cancer mortality in men and women aged 35–44 in the US between 1950 and 1999. Reproduced with permission from Deaths from Cancer.[1]

from smoking-related causes. If rates of smoking persist at current levels, half of all smokers in China will eventually be killed by smoking-related causes.

A case–control study in 16 000 cases and 16 000 controls in Southern India showed a twofold relative risk of mortality in smokers aged 25–69 years compared with non-smokers.[6] Smoking was the cause of about 60% of deaths from tuberculosis, 45% of deaths from other respiratory disorders, one-third of deaths from cancer and one-quarter of vascular deaths; overall, about one-quarter of all smokers died in middle-age.

In the USA, one million people become new smokers every year, and about half will eventually die as a result of smoking-related diseases if they continue to smoke. Eventual risks for smokers in China and India, where about 60% and about 40% of young men, respectively, smoke, will be similar. Worldwide, about 30 million people become new smokers a year – about 50% of young men and 10% of young women. With the smoking-related mortality rate standing at about 50%, if more than 20 million of these smokers fail to stop, there will be more than 10 million tobacco-related deaths per year later in this century, which is equivalent to 100 million tobacco-related deaths *per decade* – the same number of tobacco-related deaths that occurred in the whole of the 20th century. Extrapolating this throughout the century, that accounts for about 450 million deaths in the first 50 years (150 million in the first quarter and 300 million in the second quarter); if current smoking patterns continue, with 30

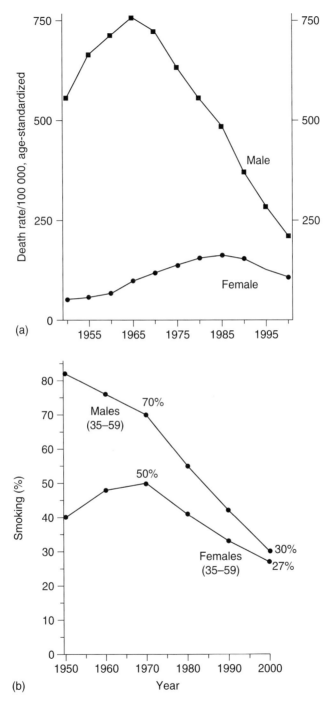

Figure 5
Cancer mortality attributed to smoking at ages 35–69 in the UK, 1950–1999 (a) and the prevalence of smoking in the UK, 1950–2000 (b).

37

million people starting to smoke and most of these continuing to smoke, the second half of the 21st century will see more than 10 million deaths per year, which is more than 100 million per decade and thus one billion deaths for the 21st century.

The proportion of people killed by smoking will not be affected much by medical progress, but would be affected by stopping smoking. Prevention of a substantial proportion of the 450 million tobacco-related deaths before 2050 requires adult cessation. Reductions in the number of children who begin smoking will prevent many deaths, but the main effects on mortality will not be seen until 2050 and later. A society that only tries to stop children from starting to smoke will lose the war against death from tobacco.

References

1. International Union Against Cancer. *Deaths from Smoking*. Geneva: International Union Against Cancer, 2006. Available at: www.deathsfromsmoking.net (last accessed 6 June 2007).
2. Doll R, Peto R, Boreham J, Sutherland I. Mortality in relation to smoking: 50 years' observations on male British doctors. *BMJ* 2004; **328**: 1519.
3. Peto R, Darby S, Deo H et al. Smoking, smoking cessation, and lung cancer in the UK since 1950: combination of national statistics with two case-control studies. *BMJ* 2000; **321**: 323–9.
4. National Center for Health Statistics. *US Mortality Public Use Data Tapes 1900–2000. US Mortality Volumes 1930–1959*. Atlanta: Centers for Disease Control and Prevention, 2003.
5. Gajalakshmi V, Peto R, Kanaka TS, Jha P. Smoking and mortality from tuberculosis and other diseases in India: retrospective study of 43 000 adult male deaths and 35 000 controls. *Lancet* 2003; **362**: 507–15.

Infection

SILVIA FRANCESCHI

In 2002, 17.7% of all cancers worldwide were attributable to infection, with infection-related cancers being more common in the developing world than in the developed world in terms of both absolute numbers and the proportion of all cancers attributable to infection (26% vs 7.7%).[1] Infective causes of cancers include:

- hepatitis viruses, which are mainly responsible for hepatocarcinomas of the liver (although some cases of non-Hodgkin lymphoma are recognized to be caused by hepatitis C virus (HCV))
- *Helicobacter pylori*, which is the main cause of cancers of the stomach and most lymphomas of the stomach
- human papillomaviruses (HPV), which cause almost all cases of cervical cancer, most cases of cancer of the anogenital tract and some cases of cancer of the neck (including 20% of oropharyngeal cancers)

Estimates of the burden of infection-related cancers are conservative for a number of reasons. Calculations of relative risks are hampered by inaccuracies in estimated prevalences of infections in patients with cancer (e.g. *H. pylori*) and in the population as whole (e.g. HCV) and, importantly, because it is not yet possible to distinguish between carcinogenic and less or non-carcinogenic strains, such as *cagA*-positive and *cagA*-negative *H. pylori*. It is also quite likely that other cancers may be associated with infections – for example, non-melanoma skin cancer is probably related to HPV, gallbladder cancer (which is common in some parts of the world) is probably related to *Helicobacter* species or *Salmonella typhi*, and the epidemiology of childhood leukaemia suggests the involvement of some infection. It would also be natural to consider a possible infective cause for colon cancer, given the enormous exposure of the colon to intestinal flora.

Hepatocellular carcinoma

Hepatitis B virus (HBV) and HCV are widely believed to cause about 20% each of cancers of the liver in developed countries, whereas in developing countries about one-third are attributed to HCV and two-thirds to HBV (Table 1).[1] A recent meta-analysis of 90 studies of

Table 1 Liver cancers attributable to hepatitis B virus (HBV) and hepatitis C virus (HCV)

Area	Cases	HBV		HCV	
		Prevalence (%)	Attributable fraction (%)	Prevalence (%)	Attributable fraction (%)
Developed countries	110 800	1.6	23.3	1.3	19.9
Developing countries	515 300	7.5	58.8	2.6	33.4
World	626 100	6.3	54.4	2.4	31.1

hepatocellular carcinoma, which included a total of 28 000 biopsies, however, found that the seroprevalence of antibody to HCV (anti-HCV) is closer to 40–50% in some European countries and slightly more than 20% even in countries with a relatively low risk of hepatitis such as the USA.[2] Surprisingly, although HBV predominates in countries such as China, Thailand and India, HCV accounts not only for the vast majority of cases of hepatocellular carcinoma in Japan (as expected) but is also more common than HBV in, for example, Mongolia and Pakistan. In addition, levels of HCV are high and increasing in Taiwan. Finally, the proportion of coinfection is high in many countries, including China and Mongolia; indeed, HCV is more often found with HBV than alone.

Despite this meta-analysis, a major problem is that data are not available for most of the world. Worryingly, data are often missing for countries adjacent to those in which HCV predominates, which suggests that the seroprevalence of HCV is very high in many countries for which data are not available. The main reason for the high prevalence of HCV is unsafe injection practice; although drug addiction is the leading factor behind such spread of HCV in a number of countries, many developing countries also have problems with unsafe injection of prescribed drugs, which are sometimes unnecessarily given parenterally when oral treatments are available. The vaccine against HBV, which has been available for some time now, has already produced great results, such as in Taiwan. Unfortunately, until a vaccine against HCV becomes available, prevention of infection with this virus is much more complicated, requiring control of blood donation, which is not yet routine in many developing countries, and education of physicians and patients to be careful not to use parenteral treatments instead of oral drugs.

In summary, the relative contribution of HCV to the current burden of liver cancer may be underestimated. Although spread of HCV has been stopped in developed countries, infection with HCV is spreading in many developing countries. In the absence of a vaccine, prevention of HCV requires an integrated strategy that involves screening of blood donations, safe injection practices and avoidance of unnecessary injections.

Gastric cancer

The leading cause of gastric cancer is infection with *H. pylori*, which results in chronic gastritis, chronic atrophic gastritis, intestinal metaplasia, dysplasia and carcinoma. Other factors that contribute to infection include lifestyle factors, particularly low intake of fresh fruit and vegetables and high intake of salt, and susceptibility factors that relate to interleukin (IL)-1β, IL-8 and other cytokines. Unfortunately, most epidemiological studies on *H. pylori* to date have been based on the detection of antibodies against the bacterium; however, this method is far from ideal in terms of sensitivity for two reasons. Firstly, it is difficult to distinguish between strains of *H. pylori* with different properties in terms of virulence and cancer-inducing power. Secondly, *H. pylori* may trigger the carcinogenetic process but may then disappear once the pH of the gastric lumen is enhanced by atrophic gastritis.

The more carcinogenic and less carcinogenic strains are best differentiated by the presence or absence of the *cagA* gene, which is a marker of the cagA pathogenicity island (cag PAI) that encodes a type IV secretion system involved in host interaction and pathogenicity. A cohort study of 2145 high-risk individuals in Venezuela used the polymerase chain reaction (PCR) to distinguish *cagA*-negative strains of *H. pylori* from *cagA*-positive strains.[3] The strength of association between the strains and the presence of infection across different degrees of gastric lesions – from normal superficial gastritis to dysplasia (cancer was not present in the population) – was strikingly different (Figure 1). *H. pylori* negative for *cagA* were associated with chronic gastritis as strongly as those positive for *cagA*, but were not associated with more severe lesions. Strains negative for *cagA* thus seem unable to induce a further progression in the carcinogenic process, whereas quite the opposite is true for *cagA*-positive strains, which produce a risk of dysplasia 16 times higher than that in uninfected individuals. Failure to distinguish *cagA*-positive from *cagA*-negative strains of *H. pylori* can thus lead to the relative risk of dysplasia being underestimated at 4.2 rather than 15.9.

A reported progressive loss of *H. pylori* as gastric atrophy develops may be an artefactual error because of the low sensitivity of older tests to detect the bacterium at the more advanced stages of disease. For example, 90% of infections in patients with dysplasia were due to *cagA*-positive strains, whereas these strains accounted for only 30% of infections in those with chronic gastritis. All stages of gastric carcinogenesis may be fostered by persistent intracellular expression of *H. pylori* virulence genes.[4,5] The fraction of gastric cancer attributable to *H. pylori* may be greater than 63%.

Cervical cancer

A meta-analysis of 14 595 biopsies of invasive cervical cancer divided according to the continent in which they were collected showed that, worldwide, 70% of cervical cancers harbour high-risk HPV-16 and -18 (which are present in the current bivalent and quadrivalent vaccines). Reassuringly, the proportion differs little across the different continents, although HPV-16 and -18 are slightly more frequent in Europe and North America (75%) than in Asia (67%) and Africa (70%) (Figure 2). Even more encouraging, however, is the fact that the eight most frequent high-risk types of HPV are virtually the same worldwide, which is promising were an octavalent vaccine to become available.

Given the importance of data on prevalence for sustaining spread of the prophylactic HPV vaccine worldwide, the International Agency for Research on Cancer (IARC) has been gathering information on the prevalence of HPV in different populations over the last 10 years. Population-based samples, which have all been tested with a sensitive, validated PCR assay in the same laboratory, have been collected from 1000–2000 women. The results shows that worldwide variation in the prevalence of high-risk HPV types is 10–20-fold, with a few countries, such as Spain and North Vietnam, having a very low prevalence but most having a prevalence of 10–15% (Figure 3). Surprisingly, the highest prevalence of high-risk HPV was found not in Africa, as was previously believed to be the case, but in Mongolia. Furthermore, the prevalence in three different areas of China (Shenzhen, Shenyang and Shanxi) was about 15%, comparable to that in India and Latin America, which contradicts the common view that China is a low-risk country for cervical cancer and suggests that the burden of cervical cancer in some provinces in China might be underestimated.

A study by Kitchener et al[6] found a much higher prevalence of high-risk HPV in young women than in middle-aged women, but the IARC's survey found that in some poor areas of

Diagnosis	cagA⁻Hp⁺/Hp⁻	cagA-negative H. pylori vs uninfected OR (95%CI)[a]	FSE[b]	OR and 95% FCI[c]	cagA⁺Hp⁻/Hp⁻	cagA-positive H. pylori vs uninfected OR (95%CI)[a]	FSE[b]	OR and 95% FCI[c]
Normal and superficial gastritis	48/27	1.00	0.242		16/27	1.00	0.320	
Chronic gastritis	532/144	2.12 (1.28–3.53)	0.096		346/144	4.33 (2.25–8.34)	0.101	
Chronic atrophic gastritis	144/58	1.44 (0.82–2.54)	0.156		124/58	3.90 (1.93–7.85)	0.160	
IM type I	166/75	1.31 (0.75–2.27)	0.141		162/75	4.14 (2.08–8.23)	0.141	
IM type II	24/10	1.46 (0.60–3.54)	0.380		53/10	10.9 (4.27–27.7)	0.349	
IM type III	15/6	1.46 (0.51–4.23)	0.484		61/6	21.9 (7.61–63.1)	0.431	
Dysplasia	18/12	0.90 (0.38–2.18)	0.375		90/12	16.0 (6.42–37.2)	0.311	

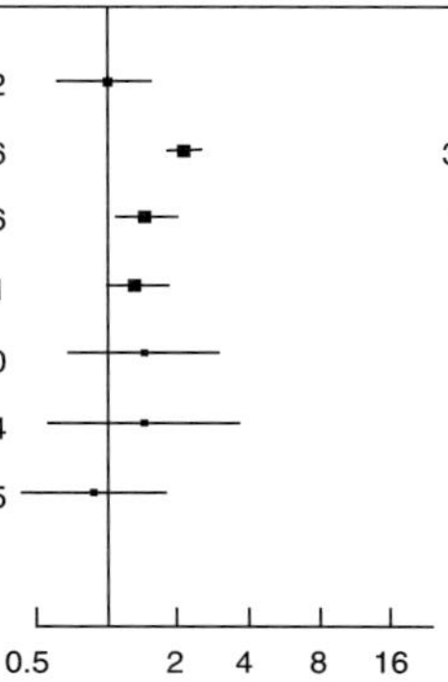

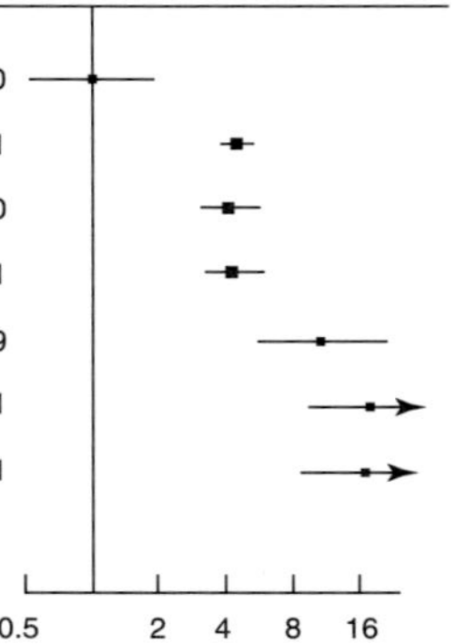

[a] Odds ratio and 95% confidence interval adjusted for age and sex
[b] Floating standard error on log scale
[c] Odds ratio and 95% floating confidence interval adjusted for age and sex

Figure 1
Odds ratios for presence of DNA from H. pylori by severity of precancerous lesions in 2145 people from Venezuela. Reproduced with permission from Plummer et al.[3]

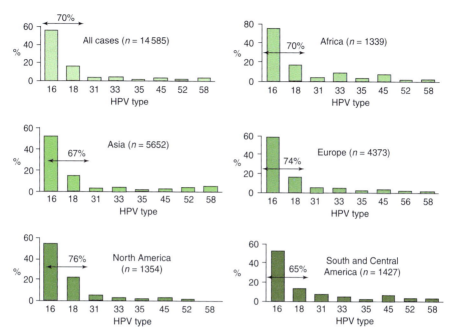

Figure 2

Prevalence of the eight most common HPV types in 14 595 cases of invasive cervical cancer by region.

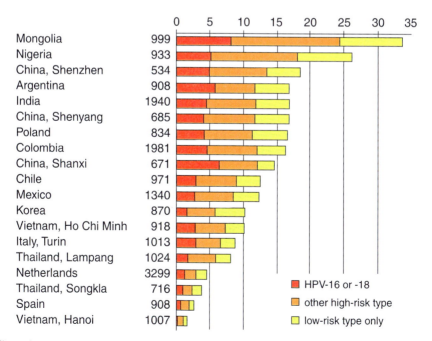

Figure 3

Prevalence of cervical HPV DNA in sexually active women aged 15–65.

Africa and Asia, young women did not have more high-risk HPV than middle-aged women. This was true regardless of the overall prevalence of HPV. Interpretation of these data is difficult, however, because the natural history of the infection is not yet understood and it is not clear whether or not natural infection causes any type-specific immunity and whether or not women can be infected, recover and be reinfected again by the same HPV type. It is clear, however, that young women in many parts of the world are not much more exposed to HPV than middle-aged women and that the age-specific prevalence of HPV must not be interpreted as the natural history of the infection, because it varies too much between populations.

HPV is covered in more detail in Professor Borysiewicz's lecture.

References

1. Parkin DM. The global health burden of infection-associated cancers in the year 2002. *Int J Cancer* 2006; **118:** 3030–44.

2. Raza SA, Clifford GM, Franceschi S. Worldwide variation in the relative importance of hepatitis B and C viruses in hepatocellular carcinoma: a systematic review. *Br J Cancer* 2007; **96:** 1127–34.

3. Plummer M, van Doorn LJ, Franceschi S, et al. *Helicobacter pylori* cytotoxin-associated genotype and gastric precancerous lesions. *J Natl Cancer Inst* 2007; in press.

4. Semino-Mora C, Doi SQ, Marty A *et al.* Intracellular and interstitial expression of *Helicobacter pylori* virulence genes in gastric precancerous intestinal metaplasia and adenocarcinoma. *J Infect Dis* 2003; **187**: 1165–77.

5. Necchi V, Candusso ME, Tava F *et al.* Intracellular, intercellular, and stromal invasion of gastric mucosa, preneoplastic lesions, and cancer by *Helicobacter pylori*. *Gastroenterology* 2007; **132**: 1009–23.

6. Kitchener HC, Almonte M, Wheeler P, et al. HPV testing in routine cervical screening: cross sectional data from the ARTISTIC trial. *Br J Cancer* 2006; **95**: 56–61.

Occupational exposure

DAVID COGGON

The International Agency for Research on Cancer (IARC) has classified 69 agents or groups of agents, 16 mixtures, and 19 exposure circumstances as group 1 carcinogens. In each of the three categories, exposure occurs principally or significantly in the workplace (22 agents or groups of agents, 5 mixtures and 17 exposure circumstances). Some carcinogens have industrial applications that depend on the properties that give rise to their carcinogenicity – for example, the ability of ethylene oxide to fumigate and sterilize depends on its capacity to damage DNA, and the ionizing properties of the radiation used in radiotherapy are what makes it useful in treatment. Most occupational carcinogens, however, occur as unwanted contaminants – for example, the presence of arsenic during the smelting of metals such as copper – or are used for purposes unrelated to their carcinogenic property – as is the case for hardwood used in the manufacture of furniture. The high proportion of established carcinogens that occur occupationally thus appears not to be a function of the types of chemicals and other agents present in the workplace, but rather a consequence of the large number of agents used in industry, the relatively high levels of occupational exposures, and the ease with which carcinogens can be identified in the workplace as compared with other settings, particularly when exposures are assessed retrospectively.

Although many carcinogens are present in the workplace, the overall burden of disease attributable to occupational exposures is smaller than for many of the cancer-causing agents discussed in other papers in this section. Precise estimates are difficult to achieve, and vary depending on whether suspected as well as definite carcinogens are included in calculations. In addition, risk differs according to the level and timing of exposure, which may vary considerably between workplaces. In 1981, Doll and Peto[1] estimated that about 4% of all cases of cancer in the USA were attributable to occupation, and a similar figure was thought to apply in the UK. The Health and Safety Executive is currently deriving a revised estimate for the UK, and although the final figure is not yet available, it is unlikely to be much higher than the 4% estimate from 1981.

Most of the known occupational carcinogens act at sites of the body with which there is direct contact (the upper and lower respiratory tract and the skin). Notable exceptions are chemicals that require metabolic activation before they can cause cancer – for example, benzene, which causes leukaemia, and some aromatic amines, which cause cancers of the urinary tract.

Occupational cancer is generally more easily preventable than cancer caused by dietary habits and other aspects of lifestyle, because legal controls can be applied to the working environment rather than relying on individuals voluntarily to change their habits on the basis of their personal assessment of risks and benefits. A well-established system with a hierarchy of interventions has evolved for the control of occupational carcinogens in the workplace. Most effective is elimination of the carcinogen altogether, which may necessitate the substitution of an alternative material. If that is not possible, engineering controls on exposure, such as local exhaust ventilation in a dusty workshop, can be instigated. This type of approach does not rely on compliance from workers, who are protected without having to take action themselves. If neither of these approaches is possible, exposure can be reduced with the use of personal protective equipment. Unfortunately, this sort of equipment is not very comfortable, can be cumbersome and can make working more difficult, which means there is a danger that workers will not fully comply with the requirements.

Two factors drive the priorities for prevention: the level of risk in the population as a whole and the attributable (absolute increase in) risk in individuals. Many occupational carcinogens do not produce a very large burden of disease at a population level – not because the risk in individuals is small but because few individuals are exposed to them. However, it is unacceptable for even a few people to be exposed to a personally high risk.

Aromatic amines

One example of a success story in the prevention of occupational cancer relates to the link between bladder cancer and aromatic amines used in the dyestuffs industry. The method that Case and colleagues used to study this in the 1950s has since been used repeatedly to investigate many other occupational carcinogens. It involved retrospectively identifying a cohort of exposed workers and then following them up to ascertain cases of cancer and assess the risk of cancer in relation to exposure.[2] Overall, Case et al found that 127 deaths from bladder cancer occurred in a cohort of workers who had been employed in the dyestuffs industry. This indicated a large increase in risk when compared with the four such deaths that would have been expected from rates in the general population. Classification of the jobs that the men had done and the chemicals to which they had been exposed allowed Case et al to show that the risk was particularly related to certain chemicals present in the industry and that one of these – β-naphthylamine (now called 2-naphthylamine) – carried an exceptionally high risk (Table 1). As a consequence of this research, the offending materials were banned and substituted with alternatives. Although concerns have been raised about other dyestuffs, workers joining the industry since the results of the study emerged have not been exposed to the carcinogens highlighted in 1954 and a major hazard has been eliminated. Unfortunately, control is not always this simple.

Table 1 *Cases of mesothelioma according to chemical. Adapted from Case et al*[2]

Exposure class	Cases	
	Observed	Expected
Aniline without magenta contact	1	0.54
Benzidine	10	0.72
α-Naphthylamine	6	0.70
β-Naphthylamine	26	0.30
All	127	4.09

Asbestos

The major burden of occupational cancer at a population level in the UK continues to arise from asbestos, the effect of which is most readily apparent in data on annual mortality from mesothelioma. This increased from 153 deaths in 1968 to almost 2000 deaths in 2001, and is still increasing.[3] This is important because controls on asbestos were introduced in the 1960s and 1970s and the problem should have been under control by now – even when the long induction period between exposure to asbestos and the development of mesothelioma is taken into account. The data suggest, however, that people continued to be exposed to asbestos, particularly in the construction industry – either because regulatory controls were inadequate or, more likely, because the enforcement of controls was unsatisfactory. Trends by birth cohort suggest that the epidemic of mesothelioma will peak between 2011 and 2015, by which time more than 2000 people will die each year from this disease.

Asbestos also causes bronchial carcinoma, but it is rather more difficult to estimate the attributable burden of cases. Some people have proposed, on the basis of findings from cohort studies, that a reasonable estimate of the burden of bronchial carcinoma can be obtained by matching it with the excess of mesothelioma cases: in other words, there is one extra carcinoma of the bronchus for each case of mesothelioma that results from exposure to asbestos. This method is unsatisfactory, however, because the excess risk of lung cancer associated with exposure to asbestos is much higher in smokers than in non-smokers, which means that the burden attributable to asbestos will decrease with the decrease in smoking rates in the population, even if there has been no reduction in exposure to asbestos. Furthermore, the relative excess of different diseases caused by asbestos may vary according to the intensity and type of asbestos to which people are exposed. Thus, the ratio of peritoneal to pleural mesothelioma varies markedly from one occupation to another, which seems to reflect differences in intensity of exposure to asbestos and in the types of asbestos fibre to which occupation are exposed.[4]

Other occupational carcinogens

Other occupational carcinogens carry nowhere near the same burden of disease at a population level as asbestos. Among the most important are polycyclic aromatic hydrocarbons, solar radiation and ionizing radiation. Polycyclic aromatic hydrocarbons occur as a consequence of combustion processes and as contaminants in various industrial materials. They can cause lung cancer if they are inhaled and historically have been a cause of skin cancer, although that risk has now largely been controlled. Solar radiation is not solely an occupational problem, but it is an important cause of non-melanoma skin cancer. Interestingly, however, melanoma is not particularly a problem in people with outdoor occupations. Ionizing radiation is a potential risk for people exposed to radon in buildings, those working in nuclear facilities, and those exposed to cosmic radiation – for example, people who fly as part of their occupation.

A number of other occupational carcinogens are less important at the population level but may still carry quite substantial risks for individuals. Exposure to dust from hardwood, which was mentioned earlier, was discovered to be a problem in the furniture industry around High

Wycombe, and excesses of sinonasal cancer in woodworkers are still recorded, particularly in those who work with hardwood. Exposure to arsenic occurs in metal smelting, and excesses of lung cancer are still seen in cohort studies of metal manufacturers. In the last 10–15 years, silica has also been noted as a cause of lung cancer; and although exposure to silica has been controlled in order to prevent silicosis, increased risks of lung cancer from exposure to silica are still recorded.

Suspected occupational carcinogens

Some agents are currently only suspected to be occupational carcinogens. For example, electromagnetic fields are suspected to cause cancer of the central nervous system, and diesel engine exhausts contain carcinogens such as polycyclic aromatic hydrocarbons. As substantial numbers of people are exposed to these potentially carcinogenic agents, even though any risks might be small at the individual level, there could be quite an important impact at a population level.

Future strategies

The main goal is to avoid another epidemic such as has been caused by exposure to asbestos. A number of approaches can be used to prevent cancer as a result of occupational carcinogens – if possible before people are exposed. Initial efforts involve trying to predict which substances are more likely to carry a risk of cancer by considering their chemical structure – for example, chemicals that can form epoxides are prone to cause cancer. In vitro and in vivo testing for genotoxicity is relatively simple. For agents for which there is a higher level of suspicion or to which people will be exposed on a very large scale, there is a case for animal carcinogenicity testing. This is more expensive, but is undertaken routinely for pesticides because they are designed to be biologically active and therefore have a higher intrinsic hazard. Although there may be a long induction period between first exposure to a carcinogen and the occurrence of a tumour, some biomarkers of cytogenetic damage may serve as an early marker of increased cancer risk, allowing more timely intervention to control exposures. Epidemiological surveillance by descriptive and analytical studies provides a final safety net, in case risks are not controlled earlier.

Summary

The workplace is an important source of risk of cancer. Occupational risks of cancer are easier to identify than many others, and generally are easier to control. The aim is to minimize risk at both a population level and an individual level. Continued vigilance is needed to control new hazards as early as possible and, if feasible, to prevent them entering the workplace at all.

References

1.   Doll R, Peto R. The causes of cancer: quantitative estimates of avoidable risks of cancer in the United States today. *J Natl Cancer Inst* 1981; **66**: 1191–308.

2.   Case RAM, Hosker ME, McDonald DB, Pearson JT. Tumours of the urinary bladder in workmen engaged in the manufacture and use of certain dyestuff intermediates in the British chemical industry. I. The role of aniline, benzidine, alpha-naphthylamine, and beta-naphthylamine. *Br J Ind Med* 1954; **11**: 75–104.

3.   Hodgson JT, McElvenny DM, Darnton AJ et al. The expected burden of mesothelioma mortality in Great Britain from 2002 to 2050. *Br J Cancer* 2005; **92**: 587–93.

4.   Coggon D, Inskip H, Winter P, Pannett B. Differences in occupational mortality from pleural cancer, peritoneal cancer and asbestosis. *Occup Environ Med* 1995; **52**: 775–7.

Discussion

DAVID COGGON, PAUL ELLIOTT, SILVIA FRANCESCHI,
RICHARD PETO, BRUCE PONDER, ELIO RIBOLI

Participant: Professor Ponder, current interventions only reduce the risk of breast cancer, could any future intervention prevent this disease?

Bruce Ponder: In terms of *BRCA1* and *BRCA2*, prevention studies based on some blockade of the action of estrogen are underway. The problem with intervention studies for women with *BRCA1* and *BRCA2*, however, is that they involve small numbers of at-risk women who must be studied for a number of years, while in the meantime more effective approaches might be conceived. A study a few years ago with an antiestrogen had to be stopped because the side-effects were too severe for the women to tolerate.

Participant: Will the UK Biobank have any impact for identifying relevant genes in studies of polygenic predisposition?

Bruce Ponder: Once the culprit genes have been identified, we will need to understand how they interact with each other and the environment, and once interactions need to be considered, statistical difficulties arise because large numbers of participants are needed. The Biobank thus could provide a well-studied set of people in whom genotyping can be undertaken and in whom the appropriate environmental information to study interactions is available, but two issues are a concern. Firstly, the Biobank may not be large enough to be adequately powered for most purposes. Secondly, for discovery and intervention, cohorts will need to be followed up annually and recalled as necessary to obtain more clinical information and samples. Unfortunately, the large cohort studies do not currently have the opportunity to recall people.

Participant: The late great Bradford Hill – the 'founder' of medical epidemiology – stated that it was a waste of time and energy exploring and disproving hypotheses that were not plausible. Professor Elliott, as radio waves are 11 orders of magnitude less than the minimum energy needed to demonstrate any biological effect, let alone produce cancer, how can you justify spending so much effort and money on exploring a hypothesis that is not merely implausible but totally impossible?

Paul Elliott: Much debate surrounds the issue of radio waves, and there are both scientific and public concerns about non-ionizing radiation and health. As it behoves epidemiologists to address public health issues, the investigation is being undertaken to answer a valid public health question. Whether or not there is a true excess that relates to a scientifically plausible hypothesis is uncertain, but the widespread exposure to this technology requires that this is properly studied to avoid potential problems in the future.

David Coggon: The energy in radiofrequency radiation is insufficient to displace electrons from their orbits, so it is not ionizing, but non-ionizing radiation can have biological effects, such as the heating effect caused by microwaves. In addition, various other biophysical mechanisms theoretically could result in biological effects from relatively low exposures to radiofrequency radiation. Although the index of suspicion is not high, there should be monitoring for possible health effects on new technologies such as mobile phones because of the enormous increase in the number of people exposed over a very short period of time.

Participant: There has been no perceptible increase in exposure to electromagnetic radiation. All biological life exists in a sea of radio waves that enter the earth's atmosphere from space, and we have all been subject to vast amounts of radio waves since the beginning of time. The tiny increase as a result of the Sutton Coldfield television mast or portable cellular telegraphy is implausibly miniscule.

Paul Elliott: The actual intensity does decrease quickly over a short distance, but it is important to consider multifactorial situations – for example, possible interactions with airborne pollutants – as it may not be the direct effect of radiation that is a concern, but perhaps indirect effects to which the radiation might contribute. Epidemiological studies aim to discover whether or not there is an excess of disease in the immediate vicinity of the transmitter.

Richard Peto: Although such studies are unlikely to reveal any new occupational carcinogens in terms of radio masts, it is better for them to be competently undertaken by epidemiologists using trusted methods than incompetently by others.

Participant: Vitamin D receptors exist all around the body – not just in the bones – and vitamin D seems to be associated with a reduced risk of cancer of the colon, although, of course, when people increase their levels of vitamin D through exposure to the sun, they might be increasing their risk of skin cancer. Professor Riboli, what is your advice to nutritionists and doctors with respect to managing the risk of cancer through diet in terms of dairy products and did you record whether people in your study ate organic or non-organic foods?

Elio Riboli: We did not collect information on consumption of organic foods in the 1990s, because organic food generally has been introduced relatively recently. The protective effect we noted for fruit, vegetables and fish was largely the result of consumption of products sold over the past 20 years, which would not have been produced through organic methods. Results on dairy products and cancer are not easy to interpret. An apparently protective effect of milk for colorectal cancer is generally thought to be due to the calcium content of milk, because clinical trials with calcium supplements have shown reduced recurrence of adenomatous polyps and a reduced risk of colon cancer. Evidence from the EPIC study suggests no link between dairy products and prostate cancer; however, two Harvard core studies have consistently shown an association. We have looked at vitamin D and meat consumption by population, and the protective effect of milk on colorectal cancer has been seen in countries where milk is and is not supplemented with vitamin D, which points to calcium as the main driver of that protective effect. Results from the EPIC study on the effects of vitamin D (more of which is obtained from sunshine in one hour than from diet in two weeks) on prostate and colorectal cancer are expected in 2008. The World Cancer Research Fund will present updated findings from their four-year evaluation of diet and cancer in November 2007.

Participant: Professor Peto, what are your thoughts regarding cancer and passive smoking.

Richard Peto: The risk of cancer is approximately proportional to the amount of smoke inhaled, so passive smoking certainly presents some risk, although the size of that risk is uncertain. The chief relevance of the restrictions on smoking to public places in the UK is likely to be the extent to which they encourage smokers to stop rather than their impact on cancers related to passive smoking.

Participant: Dr Franceschi, is it likely that all cancers will have a viral basis?

Silvia Franceschi: Epidemiological evidence for some cancers provides substantial clues – for example, cervical cancer was known to be caused by a sexually transmitted disease long before HPV was discovered. For many years, progress in this field was hampered by the lack of detection methods sensitive and accurate enough to detect the viruses or bacteria at very low copy numbers, and that is why I predict a certain expansion in the fraction of cancers attributable to infection, but I do not believe that all cancers will turn out to have a viral source.

Participant: Professor Coggon, I believe the particulates in diesel engine exhausts are very similar in size to the nanoparticles now being included in cosmetics, toiletries and other substances used by the general public. Is the safety of nanoparticles in occupational, environmental and general use being investigated?

David Coggon: The high surface area of nanoparticles relative to their mass affects their chemical properties, which also depend on the components on the surface, so we cannot assume that all nanoparticles will behave in the same way. As with mobile phones and radiofrequency radiation, nanoparticles are a rapidly expanding new technology, so their effects need to be monitored carefully. The Health and Safety Executive has identified nanotechnology as a possible source of new occupational risks to health. Initial research on the toxicology of nanoparticles is being conducted in the laboratory, where results can be obtained relatively quickly, but longer-term epidemiological studies are likely to follow.

Section Three: The Impact of Screening for Common Cancers

Prostate cancer

PETER BOYLE

A large increase in the number of cases of prostate cancer occurred between 1995 and 2002, and it is now the second most common cancer in the world. The burden of prostate cancer can be measured through data on incidence, mortality, person-years of life lost and person-years of life lost per death. In terms of incidence, data from the US National Cancer Institute's Surveillance Epidemiology and End Results (SEER) programme show that prostate cancer was the most common form of cancer in men in the USA between 1996 and 2000 (Figure 1a).[1] Mortality associated with prostate cancer was much lower than that associated with lung cancer, however, and about the same as that associated with colorectal cancer (Figure 1b). In terms of person-years of life lost, prostate cancer had a moderate effect, because it has a much higher incidence in older men than younger men (Figure 1c); for the same reason, it had the smallest effect in terms of person-years of life lost per death (Figure 1d).

Among several methods that have been proposed to screen for prostate cancer, prostate-specific antigen (PSA) testing and bone scanning diagnose the condition too late for treatment to be effective. Case–control studies have found conflicting results for digital rectal examination.

The PSA test was first approved in 1986 for the monitoring of progression in patients with prostate cancer. In 1991, William Catalona published results obtained from a large series of men in whom he measured PSA; he concluded that the screening programme identifies patients at high risk of cancer.[2] Although published in the *New England Journal of Medicine*, the study was flawed for the purposes of evaluating PSA as a screening tool, because there was no parallel control group: the study simply involved testing levels of PSA in a large series of consecutive male patients. The medical profession took the results of this paper very seriously, however, and in the two months after it was published, a 50% increase in the number of PSA tests ordered in the Seattle Puget Sound Health Maintenance Organization was recorded. The same pattern was repeated across the whole of the USA, and even some of the Harvard prospective studies showed a huge increase in the number of locally confined prostate cancers diagnosed.

Four randomized trials have investigated or are in the process of investigating the efficacy of prostate cancer screening, mainly using the PSA test. The Quebec study was claimed to be the first randomized trial to show the efficacy of screening for prostate cancer. Labrie presented the data in the plenary session at the annual meeting of the American Society of Clinical Oncology (ASCO) in Los Angeles in 1998.[3] He reported death rates of 48.7 per 100 000 in unscreened men and 15 per 100 000 in screened men, with a claimed odds ratio of 3.25 in

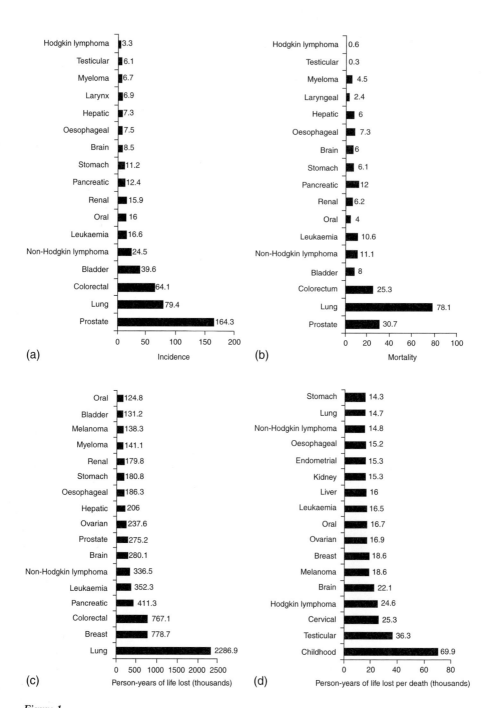

Figure 1

Incidence (a) and mortality (b) in the USA, 1996–2000, and person-years of life lost (c) and person-years of life lost per death (d) in 2000.

favour of screening. As an invited discussant, however, I re-analysed the data on an intention-to-screen basis and found a 16% excess of deaths in the group invited to screening, which suggests that the comparison of compliers with non-compliers may have been affected by selection bias. The second randomized trial to be published came from Norrköping in Sweden and had a very unusual and poor design. This study reported 292 diagnoses of prostate cancer in a control group and 82 in a screening group, with the reported rate of diagnosis claimed to be 47% higher in screened men than in controls.[4] The intention-to-screen analysis on the data, however, calculated the relative risk of death from prostate cancer to be 1.04: that is, a 4% increase in the risk of death from prostate cancer in the group offered screening. A recent Cochrane collaboration review concluded that both of these randomized trials were of poor quality and had significant limitations in their methods, and a pooled analysis produced a relative risk of death of 1.01, with a non-significant confidence interval.[5]

Results of two large randomized trials have been awaited for many years. The Prostate, Lung, Colorectal and Ovarian (PLCO) cancer trial in the USA started in 1993. It recruited 37 000 men aged 55–74 years into a screening group and the same number into a parallel control group. The European randomized study of screening for prostate cancer was started in 1991 and recruited 83 645 men aged 50–75 years into a screening group and 99 393 men into a control group. These trials have been ongoing for 14 and 17 years, respectively, without producing results on the efficacy of screening.

The PSA test itself is a simple blood test that involves minimal risk to study participants; the risk increases only when a patient is treated after receiving a diagnosis of prostate cancer. It is straightforward, cheap, readily available and easily acceptable to most men. In 1996, 83% of prostate cancer diagnoses in white men and 77% in black men were preceded by a PSA test. In 1998, the annual rate of PSA tests among Medicare beneficiaries reached 35% in white men and 25% in black men. In 2000, 12.5 million men had a PSA test in the USA. The annual number of Australian men tested increased fivefold between 1989 and 1996, 27% of men aged ≥50 years had at least one PSA test in 1995 and 1996, and 33% of men aged 60–69 years had a test in this period. In Getafe, a town in Spain close to Madrid, the rate of PSA tests was 21.6 per 1000 person-years in the general population, 86.8 per 1000 person-years in men aged 55–69 years and 152.6 per 1000 person-years in men older than 70 years. Even in Milan, Italy, where there has been no campaign to publicize or encourage prostate cancer screening, 26.9% of men aged ≥40 years without a history of prostate cancer were estimated to have received a PSA test in 1999 or 2000. In men aged ≥50 years, the rate rose to 34%.

The availability of such a simple and cheap test has given rise to some very interesting and important consequences. The first is 'contamination' in randomized trials. The sample size for a clinical trial is calculated to give the number of events required to achieve an appropriate level of statistical power. Zelen et al[6] showed that the effective sample size is equal to $n(1 - p)^2$, where p is the proportion of the control group who received the treatment and n is the original number of events required. In prostate screening trials, p would be the proportion of the control group who have their PSA measured outside the study. If the contamination rate is 10% then the effective sample size is 0.81 times the number of people in the study. The likely consequence of the high rate of PSA testing in the population is that contamination rates in clinical trials will be around 30–50%, and this is having a major impact on the effective sample size of studies; furthermore, because recruitment has long since closed, considerable delays are being encountered in acquiring enough events (deaths from prostate cancer) to make comparisons between the screened and unscreened groups.

The side-effects of radical therapy for all forms of prostate cancer have been well known for many years, so whether or not to recommend screening depends on whether any moderate reduction in mortality is offset by a decreased quality of life for the men treated. If, for example, one-third of men diagnosed with prostate cancer die from prostate cancer, there will be 1000 deaths from prostate cancer for every 3000 cases.[7] If screening were introduced and decreased mortality by 30% (a value for which there is currently no evidence), the death rate would be about 700. The incidence would double, however, so there would actually be 6000 cases of prostate cancer, most of which would be at an early stage suitable for radical therapy. In a random sample of Medicare patients in the USA, Podolski found a rate of serious adverse events (30-day postoperative mortality, incontinence, wearing pads at 6 months or a year, and an unchangeable loss of potency) of 28.6% in those treated radically. This means that if 4000 of the 6000 patients were treated radically, 1114 serious adverse events would be expected. The prevention of one death thus could result in serious adverse events in 2–3 men. Although a treatment needs to be in place for all men in the community, it could lead to a situation in which a huge loss in quality of life more than offsets a moderate reduction in mortality through screening. Even if the results of ongoing trials are null or inconclusive, however, it is clear that nothing can stop the inexorable rise in the use of PSA testing in the community. It would be helpful at this point, therefore, to introduce some method of evaluating the outcome of such an activity in a scientifically meaningful manner.

Nerve-sparing radical prostatectomy was introduced to the federal state of the Tyrol, Austria, in 1998. Unorganized cancer detection began in 1990, and PSA testing was made freely available to every man aged 45–75 years in 1993. In the first full year in which this offer was made, 32% of men in the defined age range were screened. By the end of the period 1995–2005, 86.6% of men who had passed through the age window had been screened at least once and 14000 had been screened 14 times. As this was a demonstration project in a community rather than a randomized trial, new ideas on how to treat and detect prostate cancer were incorporated into the algorithm and used throughout the state. Men in the rest of Austria were not offered PSA testing. Using the standardized mortality rate with the pre-screening era (1986–90) used as a baseline; the rate in 1991 was 113% of baseline, but this has gradually reduced to just 46% of baseline in 2005. In the rest of Austria, a gradual evolution in the uptake of PSA (as in most countries) has been accompanied by a 3% annual reduction in mortality since 1993 (similar to the reduction in the USA), while a 7.2% reduction was observed in the Tyrol. Reassuringly, the screening did not result in a deferral of prostate cancers until after the age of 80 years, as there was a reduction of 64% in the number of cancer deaths expected in the Tyrol and 93% in the rest of Austria. When the age-standardized mortality was analysed with a different smoothing trend, a larger and more rapid reduction was seen in the Tyrol than in the rest of Austria. The entire state of the Tyrol has outstanding urological services for every patient, with free immediate access to many different types of treatment. A study of morbidity and mortality after radical prostatectomy in a series of 1663 patients in 1998–2004 showed no mortality at 30 days, no ureteral injury, and incidences of 0.6% for rectal injury (which has decreased to 0.1% since 2000), 0.7% for rectal bleeding that required intervention, 80.6% for continence at 3 months and 95.1% for continence at 12 months.

Since 2000, the potency rate has improved to 78.9% in 512 men younger than 65 years. Overall, these results confirm that, in the best of circumstances, PSA testing can be effective.

A paradox seen in many studies in the USA is that men diagnosed with prostate cancer live as long as, or longer than, men who have not been given such a diagnosis. Walsh and Thompson[8] sought an explanation for this paradox by studying a consecutive series of surgical patients treated at the Veterans Association Hospital in San Antonio. After surgery, 72% of men had a change of medical regimen, 61% had a change of drug treatment and 29% received a new medical diagnosis. Walsh and Thompson proposed that changes of such magnitude would be expected to affect survival outcomes of men recently diagnosed with prostate cancer.

Since the introduction of PSA testing, the reported incidence of low-grade prostate cancer has declined. A population-based cohort of 1858 prostate cancers diagnosed during 1990–92 was assembled at the Connecticut cancer registry.[9] Histological slides were reread between 2002 and 2004 by an experienced prostate pathologist blinded to the original Gleason scores.

Worryingly, the contemporary Gleason score readings were significantly higher than the original readings (the mean score increased from 5.95 to 6.8). The contemporary Gleason score-standardized mortality for prostate cancer (1.50 deaths per 100 person-years) seemed to be 28% lower than the standardized historical rate (2.08 deaths per 100 person-years), even though the overall outcome was unchanged. The authors concluded that the decline in reported incidence of low-grade prostate cancers seems to be the result of reclassification of Gleason scores over the past decade, which resulted in an apparent improvement in clinical outcome.

In a cohort of 597 642 men aged ≥70 years assembled from 104 US Veterans Hospitals during 2002 and 2003, 56% of elderly men had a PSA test in 2003: 64% in men aged 70–74 years and 36% among men aged ≥85 years.[10] The US Preventive Services Task Force noted that screening tests can detect prostate cancer at an earlier stage than clinical detection and that one study provides good evidence that radical prostatectomy reduces disease-specific mortality in localized disease.[11] They also claimed that men with a life expectancy of less than 10 years are unlikely to benefit from screening even under favourable assumptions, concluding that: 'although potential harms of screening for prostate cancer can be established, the presence or magnitude of potential benefits cannot. Therefore, the net benefit of screening cannot be determined.' They recommend that if physicians opt to perform screening for individual patients, they should first discuss uncertain benefits and possible harms. The American Medical Association believes that launching mass prostate screening programmes is premature at this time and also recommends that physicians should provide patients with information regarding the risks and benefits so that they can make an informed decision about screening. Furthermore, when screening is done, it should include both a PSA blood test and digital rectal examination, and men most likely to benefit include those who have a life expectancy of at least 10 years, those who are ≥40 years and of African-American descent, those who have an affected first-degree relative, and others who are ≥50 years.

Shared decision making has its problems, however. Merenstein was sued for letting a patient decide whether to be screened for prostate cancer after engaging him in shared decision making, as current guidelines recommend.[12] The patient declined screening, was later found to have prostate cancer and successfully sued the practice. Merenstein was eventually exonerated, but his residency programme was found liable for teaching him to engage patients in shared decision making to decide whether to test for prostate cancer

The real impact and tragedy of prostate cancer screening is the doubling of the lifetime risk of a diagnosis of prostate cancer without any effect on the risk of dying from this disease. In 1985, an American man had an 8.7% lifetime risk of being diagnosed with prostate cancer and a 2.5% risk of dying from prostate cancer.[13] Twenty years later, in 2005, an American man had a 17% lifetime risk of being diagnosed with prostate cancer and a 3% risk of dying from prostate cancer.[14] Despite this, the increase in PSA testing will be impossible to stop. Trial results for and against testing have always been contentious among supporters and opponents of screening. In the case of breast cancer, even with data available from nine randomized trials with reasonable methods, claims have been made that there is no evidence to support mammographic screening. With fewer trials available for evaluating prostate cancer screening and with contamination rates in the control group likely to be very high, questions will undoubtedly be posed about the reliability of the findings.

Conclusion

Evidence shows harms of screening, but no evidence from randomized trials shows efficacy of prostate cancer screening with PSA. Population screening for prostate cancer cannot be recommended at present. Testing for PSA and integrated programmes of multidisciplinary diagnosis and treatment are effective at reducing mortality from prostate cancer. The availability of a cheap and safe test such as PSA has thrown up new issues and challenges.

References

1. US National Cancer Institute: Surveillance Epidemiology and End Results. www.seer.cancer.gov
2. Catalona WJ, Smith DS, Ratliff TL et al. Measurement of prostate-specific antigen in serum as a screening test for prostate cancer. *N Engl J Med* 1991; **324**: 1156–61.
3. Labrie F, Dupont A, Candas B et al. Decrease of prostate cancer death by screening: first data from the Quebec prospective and randomized study. *Proc Am Soc Clin Oncol* 1998; **17**: Abst 4.
4. Sandblom G, Varenhorst E, Löfman O et al. Clinical consequences of screening for prostate cancer: 15 years follow-up of a randomised controlled trial in Sweden. *Eur Urol* 2004; **46**: 717–23.
5. Ilic D, O'Connor D, Green S, Wilt T. Screening for prostate cancer. *Cochrane Database Syst Rev* 2007; (2): CD004720.
6. Zelen M, Parker RA. Case–control studies and Bayesian inference. *Stat Med* 1986; **5**: 261–9.
7. Boyle P. Screening for prostate cancer: have you had your cholesterol measured? *BJU Int* 2003; **92**: 191–9.
8. Walsh RM, Thompson IM. Prostate cancer screening and disease management: how screening may have an unintended effect on survival and mortality – the camel's nose effect. *J Urol* 2007; **177**: 1303–6.
9. Albertsen PC, Hanley JA, Barrows GH et al. Prostate cancer and the Will Rogers Phenomenon. *J Natl Cancer last* 2005; **97**: 1248–53.
10. Walter LC, Bertenthal D, Lindquist K, Konety BR. PSA screening among elderly men with limited life expectancies. *JAMA* 2006; **296**: 2336–42.
11. Harris R, Lohr KN. Screening for prostate cancer: an update of the evidence for the U.S. Preventive Services Task Force. *Ann Intern Med* 2002; **137**: 917–29.
12. Merenstein D. Winners and losers. *JAMA* 2004; **291**: 15–16.

13. Seidman H, Mushinski MH, Gelb SK, Silverberg E. Probabilities of eventually developing or dying of cancer – United States, 1985. *CA Cancer J Clin* 1985; **35**: 36–56.

14. Jemal A, Siegel R, Ward E, Murray T, Xu J, Thun MJ. Cancer statistics, 2007. *CA Cancer J Clin* 2007; **57**: 43–66.

Colorectal cancer

WENDY ATKIN

The case in the UK for a screening programme for colorectal cancer is strong, as it is the second most common cause of death from cancer – exceeding deaths from breast and cervical cancer, for which there are well-established screening programmes.[1] Colorectal cancer is expensive to manage, with NHS expenditure exceeding £500 million per year for imaging, hospital stays, surgery, the increasing costs of radiotherapy and adjuvant chemotherapy, and palliative care. Incidence rates have increased very little; however, the numbers of cases diagnosed each year are due to increase dramatically to a predicted 50 000 cases by 2025 due to an aging population, and this will dramatically increase the costs associated with this disease.

The causes of the disease are related to a sedentary lifestyle and a typically Western, high-calorie diet based on meat and little dietary fibre. However a method of primary prevention in middle age has proved elusive, and it seems likely that a low-risk lifestyle needs to be maintained from early in life to have any impact on incidence.

Mortality has been decreasing over the past few years, but survival is still less than 50%. Although new treatment methods are available, treatment is only marginally effective once the disease has reached advanced stages. A more effective method of reducing mortality rates is by early detection through screening. The major risk factor for colorectal cancer is older age, and there are no other risk factors in 75% of cases, so screening has to be offered to the whole population. Although screening programmes are very costly, savings could be made through avoided treatment costs.

Early detection

Early detection of cancer has been the traditional approach to reducing mortality from colorectal cancer, as localized disease has a high survival rate (exceeding 80%), whereas disease that has spread beyond the bowel wall has lower survival rates (Figure 1). Some cases are indolent and diagnosed symptomatically at the early stage. However, most colorectal cancers that are advanced at diagnosis were asymptomatic during the early, localized stage. The challenge of screening is to detect cancers destined to be more advanced at diagnosis while they are still localized (Figure 2). Screening can therefore only be effective if the progression from a localized to an advanced cancer is sufficiently slow to allow detection of localized cancers through screening at intervals long enough to be cost-effective. Trials have confirmed that this is indeed the case for colorectal cancer.

In contrast to some cancers, such as breast cancer, colorectal cancer has a visible pre-invasive phase. Cross-sectional studies show that most, although possibly not all, colorectal cancers arise from precancerous lesions called adenomas, which are generally asymptomatic. These

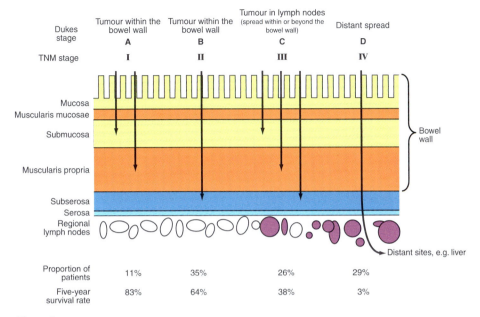

Figure 1
Colorectal cancer: modified Dukes and TNM stage and 5-year survival rate.

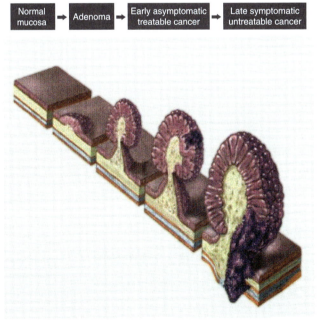

Figure 2
Scientific rationale for screeening.

tend to be polypoid and detectable endoscopically, so that cancers could potentially be prevented through the detection and removal of adenomas.

Different screening tests detect different stages of the disease. Whether the screening test detects early localized cancer or the premalignant adenoma has some implications. Detecting cancer at an early stage can reduce mortality, as has been confirmed in trials, but it does not have any effect on incidence or morbidity, because even early cancers usually need some form of surgery. In fact, early detection will allow surgery to be avoided in only about 5% of cancers. The time for progression of an asymptomatic early treatable cancer to a symptomatic late and untreatable carcinoma is also believed to be just 2–3 years (see Figure 2), so that detection of early cancer requires frequent testing – every 2 years is believed to be the maximum interval. Early detection of cancer through screening is also costly, because the cost of screening must be added to the cost of managing the cancers detected by screening. Furthermore, positive tests for cancer cause anxiety to the patient. Screening that detects adenomas aims to decrease mortality through a reduction in incidence and morbidity. As adenomas take a long time to become malignant, the screening interval could be very infrequent and the screening costs could be offset against avoided treatment costs, Furthermore, if the population understands that the test is not screening for cancer but aims to prevent cancer, anxiety levels would be lower.

A variety of different methods for colorectal cancer screening have been available for the last decade, and the choice may have resulted in a delay in the introduction of a screening programme in the UK. The numerous options potentially suitable for screening include:

- endoscopy (flexible sigmoidoscopy and colonoscopy)
- imaging (barium enema and computed tomographic colonography)
- stool tests (guaiac faecal occult blood tests, immunochemical faecal occult blood tests and molecular markers)
- blood tests (molecular markers)

NHS Bowel Cancer Screening Programme

The NHS Bowel Cancer Screening Programme was introduced to the UK in 2006. The programme in England invites people aged 60–69 years at intervals of 2 years, while Scotland and Wales intend to include a wider age-range of 50–74 years. The programme is based on the guaiac faecal occult blood test, which costs only €1 (equivalent to £0.68 per set of tests). Because blood is not spread uniformly and bleeding is thought to be intermittent and at low levels, the test has to be repeated three times using samples from two different parts of the stool. When the test is developed, it produces a clear positive, equivocal or negative result. People with a positive guaiac test will undergo examination of the colon, using colonoscopy, to confirm the test's positive findings. Currently, about 1 in 10 people with a positive guaiac test will be found to have cancer. In successive rounds of tests, the rate is about 1 in 20. This test was chosen because three large trials have shown a modest but significant and consistent 16% reduction in mortality.[2-4] As expected, the test has no effect on incidence, because adenomas do not usually bleed.

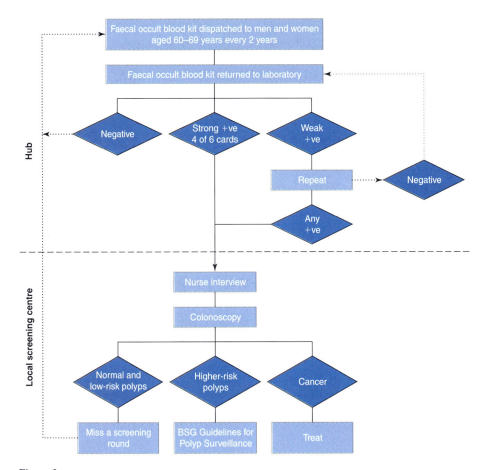

Figure 3
Screening pathway in the NHS Colorectal Cancer Screening Programme.

The infrastructure required for the screening programme is another reason for the delay in its introduction. The programme comprises five hubs, each of which serves 10 million of the English population and about 20 screening centres that investigate the people who test positive on the guaiac test. The hub is responsible for dispatching and developing the test kits and informing screening centres about people who tested positive during screening. In the current English protocol (Figure 3), people with four positive cards of six are considered positive, while those with fewer positive cards are considered weakly positive and undergo repeat testing. A nurse interviews people who test positive and colonoscopy is performed within 2 weeks. Those with a negative colonoscopy return to the screening programme, those with cancer are referred to the multidisciplinary team, and those with intermediate or high-risk polyps enter a surveillance programme (Figure 4).[5]

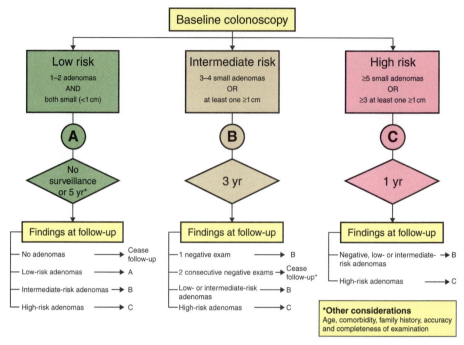

Figure 4

*Surveillance following adenoma removal. Reproduced from Atkin WS, Saunders BP; British Society for Gastroenterology; Association of Coloproctology for Great Britain and Ireland. Surveillance guidelines after removal of colorectal adenomatous polyps. Gut 2002; **51** (Suppl 5): v6–9.*[5]

Endoscopic screening

Endoscopic screening is an alternative method that is able to detect polyps (precursor adenomas). Colonoscopy examines the whole colon, while flexible sigmoidoscopy examines only the distal part – the sigmoid colon and rectum. A person prepares for a flexible sigmoidoscopy at home by using an enema an hour before coming into the unit, and this seems to be acceptable to the population in the UK.[6] The procedure itself takes 4 minutes – or 8 minutes if polyps are found and removed during the procedure. This approach aims to reduce the number of people who need a colonoscopy, which involves complete bowel preparation with 12–18 hours of dietary restriction and laxatives, and often requires sedation. Colonoscopy is a much bigger procedure than flexible sigmoidoscopy and is not recommended for population screening in the UK, although it is recommended in the USA and in the UK for people with a strong family history of colorectal cancer.

Flexible sigmoidoscopy is a relatively cheap procedure that costs only about £80. Studies have shown that it is feasible for implementation in a screening programme, but insufficient evidence of effectiveness is available to recommend its use at present, as the only studies are epidemiological, and cohort and case–control studies are subject to bias. Encouragingly, however, all studies to date seem to consistently show a 60–80% reduction in the development of cancers within reach of the sigmoidoscope and a long duration of protection in the region of

10–15 years.[7] Indeed, sigmoidoscopy may need to be offered only once:[8] although the incidence of distal colorectal cancer increases throughout life, the prevalence of adenomas seems to plateau at the age of 60 years. This suggests that anyone who is going to have a distal adenoma would have developed it by the age of 60 years and that most distal cancers develop from adenomas that developed before that age. Interestingly, this does not happen in the proximal colon, where the prevalence of adenomas increases throughout life without any discernable plateau.

Four randomized trials are ongoing. The UK Flexible Sigmoidoscopy (Flexi-Scope) trial started in 1994 and screened 40 000 people (see below). The Prostate, Lung, Colorectal and Ovarian (PLCO) cancer trial, which started in 1992 and did not finish recruiting until 2001, is not expected to report until 2015. Unfortunately, the level of exposure to screening in the USA (as a result of their national recommendations) will make it hard to identify the true benefit of the screening. This is not a problem for the Flexi-Scope trial, as exposure to sigmoidoscopy in the UK is still low and the faecal occult blood test used in the Bowel Cancer Screening Programme is not able to detect high rates of adenomas. The Sigmoidoscopy for Colorectal Cancer (SCORE) study undertaken in Northern Italy used the protocol from the UK (see below) and is also expected to analyse its results next year. A similar study (NORCAPP) was undertaken in Norway more recently.

Flexi-Scope trial

The protocol for the Flexi-Scope trial, which is in line with the protocol likely to be introduced nationally in the UK, involves giving a single flexible sigmoidoscopy at about the age of 55–60 years and removing all small polyps during the procedure. Colonoscopy is reserved for people with large polyps that cannot be removed during flexible sigmoidoscopy or polyps that confer an increased risk of developing more advanced adenomas or cancer (around 5%). The baseline results were published in 2002.[9] Contrary to expectation, the results suggested that flexible sigmoidoscopy could be implemented nationally, because it is quick, people are prepared to take an enema, rates of detection of adenomas are high (particularly in men), cancers are detected earlier even than with faecal occult blood testing and it is safe.

The trial is due to be analysed in 2008. A long follow-up period is necessary, as, although the study is intended to show a reduction in the incidence of cancer, screening identifies prevalent cancers, so the study began with more cancers in the intervention group; however, removal of adenomas is expected to prevent cancers. The study has been running for about 8 years and the magnitude of observed benefit is predicted to be increasing year on year. Whether the effect of a single sigmoidoscopy lasts forever, as has been hypothesized, is uncertain and is one of the questions to be answered by the trial.

A recent analysis by the Department of Health indicated that, by preventing cancers, flexible sigmoidoscopy at the age of 55 or 60 years could result in a possible saving of £12 for every person screened (if the assumptions, on which all cost-effectiveness models depend, are correct).[10] The study also noted that it would be expensive to undertake faecal occult blood testing for two decades from the age of 50 years but a lot less costly if testing were undertaken for just one decade; indeed, the latter approach was shown to be more equitable, because sufficient colonoscopy facilities would be available throughout the country to implement this approach nationwide. The decision was taken to use this approach initially in the colorectal cancer screening programme offering screening to people aged 60–69 years. Once it is implemented in this narrow age range across the nation, a decision will be made on whether to increase the age range, introduce flexible sigmoidoscopy at the start of screening or consider a different screening technology.

Rates of colorectal cancer in the USA have been decreasing over the last few years (Figure 5), possibly because of the widespread use of colonoscopy and sigmoidoscopy. Interestingly, the incidence has only been decreasing in cancers of the distal colon, with little change in incidence in cancers of the proximal colon, even though colonoscopy is the main procedure used.[11,12] The reduction is less marked in women, apparently because men are much more likely to attend endoscopic screening than women. The reason for this is not clear, although women are more likely to attend for examination when the procedure is to be undertaken by a woman. As a result, the effectiveness of nurse endoscopists, most of whom are women, has been investigated. Several studies have shown that nurses are as good as doctors at performing flexible sigmoidoscopy and identifying polyps.

Flexible sigmoidoscopy is criticized in the USA for preventing cancers only in half of the colon and has been likened to mammography of just one breast.[13] The comparison is inappropriate, however, as it assumes that the proximal and distal (right-sided and left-sided) colon are equally accessible and that colonoscopy and sigmoidoscopy are similar procedures. In reality, as a first-line mass screening test, colonoscopy fails on manpower, acceptability, safety and efficacy. Specialist nurses would be unable to undertake screening colonoscopy, as it takes much more skill than sigmoidoscopy and the manpower simply is not available. Acceptability is also a problem for colonoscopy, and even in the USA uptake is low. The risks for

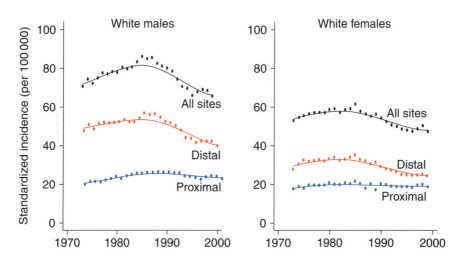

Figure 5

Trends in the incidence of colorectal cancer in the USA. Data from the US National Cancer Institute's Surveillance Epidemiology and End Results programme. Courtesy of Andrew Renehan.

colonoscopy are greater, since the wall in the top of the colon is thinner, which increases the risk of perforation when removing polyps. Finally, colonoscopy appears to have only limited ability to prevent proximal colon cancer, and, as described earlier, colonoscopy in the USA has so far had little impact on rates of proximal colon cancer while rates of distal cancer are falling (see Figure 5). This may be because colonoscopy is technically difficult and many endoscopists are unable to give a complete examination of the proximal colon. It may be because the biology and epidemiology of proximal colon cancer is different and requires a different screening approach.

The challenge now is to ensure that the NHS Bowel Cancer Screening Programme is a success, with high uptake rates and a significant effect on colorectal cancer mortality rates. The results of the clinical trials of flexible sigmoidoscopy may provide new opportunities for colorectal cancer prevention. The challenge will then be to find a cost-effective method of preventing proximal colon cancer.

References

1. http://info.cancerresearchuk.org/cancerstats.

2. Hardcastle JD, Chamberlain JO, Robinson MH et al. Randomised controlled trial of faecal-occult-blood screening for colorectal cancer. *Lancet* 1996; **348**: 1472–7.

3. Kronborg O, Fenger C, Olsen J et al. Randomised study of screening for colorectal cancer with faecal-occult-blood test. *Lancet* 1996; **348**: 1467–71.

4. Mandel JS, Bond JH, Church TR et al. Reducing mortality from colorectal cancer by screening for fecal occult blood. Minnesota Colon Cancer Control Study. *N Engl J Med* 1993; **328**: 1365–71.

5. Atkin WS, Saunders BP; British Society for Gastroenterology; Association of Coloproctology for Great Britain and Ireland. Surveillance guidelines after removal of colorectal adenomatous polyps. *Gut* 2002; **51**(Suppl 5): v6–9.

6. Atkin WS, Hart A, Edwards R et al. Single blind, randomised trial of efficacy and acceptability of oral picolax versus self administered phosphate enema in bowel preparation for flexible sigmoidoscopy screening. *BMJ* 2000; **320**: 1504–8.

7. Selby JV, Friedman GD, Quesenberry CP, Weiss NS. A case–control study of screening sigmoidoscopy and mortality from colorectal cancer. *N Engl J Med* 1992; **326**: 653–7.

8. Atkin W, Cuzick J, Northover J, Whynes D. Prevention of colorectal cancer by once-only sigmoidoscopy. *Lancet* 1993; **341**: 736–40.

9. UK Flexible Sigmoidoscopy Screening Trial Investigators. Single flexible sigmoidoscopy screening to prevent colorectal cancer: baseline findings of a UK multicentre randomised trial. *Lancet* 2002; **359**: 1291–300.

10. Tappenden P, Chilcott J, Eggington S et al. Option appraisal of population-based colorectal cancer screening programmes in England. *Gut* 2007; **56**: 677–84.

11. Chu KC, Tarone RE, Chow WH et al. Temporal patterns in colorectal cancer incidence, survival, and mortality from 1950 through 1990. *J Natl Cancer Inst* 1994; **86**: 997–1006.

12. Cress RD, Morris C, Ellison GL, Goodman MT. Secular changes in colorectal cancer incidence by subsite, stage at diagnosis, and race/ethnicity, 1992–2001. *Cancer* 2006; **107**(Suppl): 1142–52.

13. Bhattacharya I, Sack EM. Screening coloroscopy: the cost of common sense. *Lancet* 1996; **347**: 1744–5.

Breast cancer

MICHAEL MICHELL

The NHS Breast Cancer Screening Programme was set up in 1989 with the aim of decreasing deaths from breast cancer by detecting, diagnosing and treating cancers when they are small and there is less risk of metastatic spread. The programme originally invited women aged 50–64 years for single-view screening every 3 years. The UK now has 90 programmes, the current revenue cost is about £70 million per annum, the age of invitation has been extended to invite women aged 50–70 years (with open access for women older than 70 years) and two-view screening, which has been shown to increase the sensitivity significantly, is now used.

Just over two million women a year are invited, with more than 1.6 million women attending screening. Uptake is reasonably good for a national screening programme, with a relatively constant average level of 74–75% since the programme started. Uptake is variable across the country, however, with a much lower uptake in London and other inner city areas – uptake in some areas of southeast London is less than 50%. This is a difficult problem to overcome and is probably multifactorial, reflecting mobility of the population, inaccuracy of records, ethnic diversity, cultural and religious issues, and language barriers (about 250 languages are currently spoken in London).

In 2004–05, the screening programme diagnosed 13 812 cases of breast cancer (about one-third of all cases in England). Around 10 940 of these were invasive, most were small (<15 mm in diameter) and 75–77% were lymph node-negative. Conservative breast-saving surgery was undertaken in 71% of patients. Ductal carcinoma accounted for about 20% of cancers found (n = 2872) and around 70% of cases were treated with conservative surgery.

The increased numbers of women who are being screened has created a capacity issue, but the programme aims to maintain the 3-year screening interval. Screening is being implemented for women in high-risk groups because of their family history and/or the presence of high-risk genes. Uptake needs to be improved, particularly in inner city areas, and a further age extension – possibly inviting women up to the age of 76 years – is under consideration. All of this will involve a large amount of work, however, which means that digital technology and new techniques will need to be implemented.

Effectiveness of breast cancer screening

Screening for breast cancer has had a mixed press over the years, and the public and members of the health profession could be forgiven for being uncertain about its effectiveness. Epidemiologically, screening is based on the fact that cancers found at an early stage will have better outcomes. A number of large-scale trials have been carried out in Europe and the USA. The Swedish Two-Counties Trial was perhaps the best conducted, and showed divergence between the control group not invited for screening and the group invited for mammographic screening (Figure 1).[1] This divergence persisted (as was also the case for colorectal cancer; see

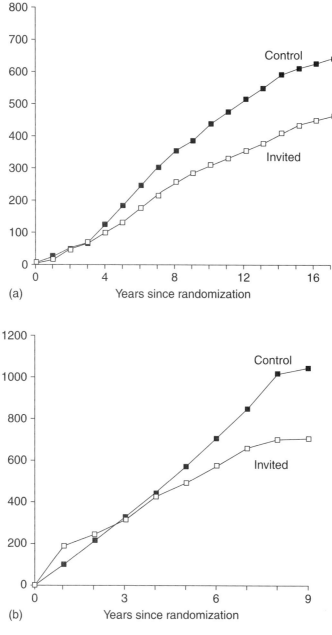

Figure 1
Cumulative mortality (a) and incidence of breast carcinoma ≥stage II (b) in invited and control groups of women aged 40–74 years in the Two-County Trial in Sweden.[1]

Trial	Enrollment (years/age)	Intervention (Invitations to screening)	Population ×1000 (screened/control)	Breast cancer mortality per 100 000 person–years (number) (screened/control)		Relative risk (95% confidence interval)
Malmö I, Sweden	1976–78/50–69	4 in 8 years	16.8/16.8	47 (134)/57 (162)		0.84 (0.68–1.04)
Kopparberg, Swedish Two-county	1976–78/50–69	3 in 6 years	23.3/10.7	20 (93)/39 (83)		0.52 (0.39–0.70)
Östergötland, Swedish Two-county	1978–81/50–69	4 in 8 years	23.6/22.4	33 (117)/40 (137)		0.81 (0.64–1.03)
Stockholm, Sweden	1981–83/50–64	2 in 4 years	24.8/13.0	14 (48)/21 (37)		0.68 (0.44–1.04)
Göteborg, Sweden	1982–84/50–59	3 in 5 years	10.1/16.0	31 (40)/33 (67)		0.94 (0.62–1.43)
Finland	1987–89/50–64	2 in 4 years	89.9/68.9	16 (64)/21 (63)		0.76 (0.53–1.09)
All trials			**188.5/147.8**	**25 (496)/36 (549)**		**0.75 (0.67–0.85)**
					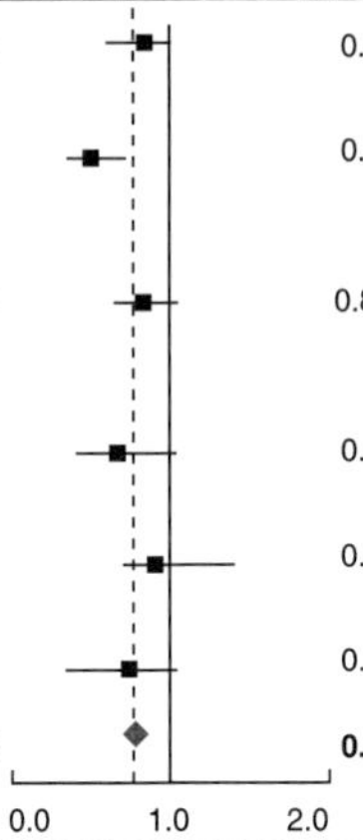 0.0 1.0 2.0	

Tests for heterogeneity between trials χ^2_5 = 8.83; $p > 0.1$; not significant

Figure 2
Efficacy of screening for breast cancer by mammography alone in women aged 50–69 years.[2]

Professor Atkin's chapter in these proceedings) and was mirrored by the decreased numbers of advanced cancers in the group invited for screening.

In a meta-analysis of all evidence available from randomized trials, the International Agency for Research on Cancer (IARC) showed a 25% reduction in mortality for women invited for screening (Figure 2). The reduction in mortality would, of course, be expected to be higher for women who attend screening regularly. The screening programme saves an estimated 1400 lives each year in England, at a cost of £3000 per year of life saved.[3] Overall, about 6 in every 1000 women aged 50–69 years will die of breast cancer in the next 10 years without screening. Screening reduces this to 4 in every 1000 women, which means that 1 in every 500 women screened is saved.

The incidence of breast cancer has been increasing steadily in the UK (with a larger increase in the early 1990s because of implementation of the screening programme). At the same time, however, the age-standardized death rate decreased by around 33%, with a steady decline in all age groups from the early 1990s.

In 1971–73, the 5-year survival rate was about 52%; this had improved to 80% by 2001–03. Interestingly, survival rates at 5, 10, 15 and 20 years were higher for women aged 50–69 years than for younger or older women.[4] Local control, surgery, radiotherapy and the implementation and additional use of systemic treatment (both hormonal therapy and chemotherapy) have certainly had an effect. The stage of diagnosis has also been brought forward by screening and perhaps because women are presenting earlier as a result of widespread publicity about breast screening and breast disease in general. Figure 3 shows an increase in stage I and

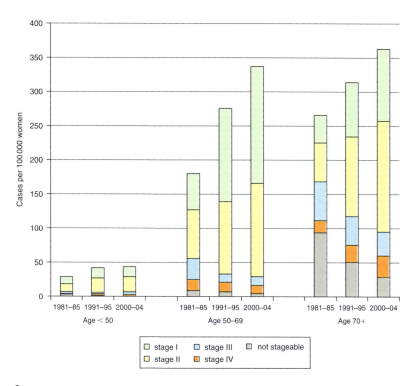

Figure 3
Rates of breast cancer in women in East Anglia by stage at diagnosis in the last three decades (Greenberg D, unpublished data, 2007).

II cancers but a corresponding decrease in later-stage cancers, certainly in the screening age group and possibly in the older age group. Encouragingly, the number with insufficient information for staging has decreased recently (Greenberg D, unpublished data, 2007).

Quality assurance is relied on to maximize the benefits (saving the lives of women with breast cancer, allowing less radical treatment and improving diagnostic services) and minimize the adverse effects of screening (anxiety, discomfort, benign biopsy and overdiagnosis). The breast screening programme in the UK has successfully implemented rigorous quality assurance – not just in terms of the technical quality of the images but also for radiologists, surgeons and every profession involved in the screening process. The programme has a good structure, with clear leadership, representation of all involved professions and a clear line of communication between the Department of Health and regional quality assurance networks. This has been underpinned by a network of national specialist training centres that offer training in every aspect of the screening process.

The standardized detection ratio shows that the sensitivity for detection of cancer has approximately doubled between 1990–91 and 2004–05. Preoperative diagnosis of cancer has also improved – in the mid-1990s, many women underwent diagnostic surgery followed by multiple operations; a positive diagnosis is now made in 90% of women with screen-detected cancers. Sophisticated diagnostic tools, such as the positive predictive referral model, have been developed to manage varying performance between different units in the country.

Conclusion

Screening has stimulated a great deal of research not only into screening but also into aspects of pathology, natural history and treatment of breast cancer. Much work is being done on technical developments, and it may be possible to use computers to read mammographic films in the future. The increased quantity of work as a result of increased numbers of women attending screening has necessitated the development of a team to cope with increased capacity; this involves a four-tier system in which assistant practitioners (non-radiographers) are being trained to take the mammograms, and radiographers are being trained to read films and to perform other tasks. Data suggest very little difference between the performance of trained radiographers and radiology film readers. Advanced practitioners in the programme are now performing tasks such as reading films, performing ultrasound of the breast, needle biopsy and wire localization. The programme provides a good example of the successful development of the team to provide additional capacity without losing quality. In the words of Professor Blamey, who believed all women with breast cancer owe screening a debt for raising standards in treatment and care: 'Getting the entire process of specialization in breast cancer and setting audit standards in breast cancer on the back of it are two of the great successes of the whole screening story. The care of breast cancer patients has improved enormously and of course the mortality is falling sharply as well.'[5]

References

1. Duffy SW, Tabar L, Vitak B et al. The Swedish Two-County Trial of mammographic screening: cluster randomisation and end point evaluation. *Ann Oncol* 2003; **14**: 1196–8.
2. International Agency for Research on Cancer/World Health Organization. *Breast Cancer Screening* (IARC Handbooks of Cancer Prevention, Vol 7). Lyon: IARC Press, 2002.
3. Advisory Committee on Breast Cancer Screening. *Screening for Breast Cancer in England: Past and Future.* Sheffield: NHS Breast Cancer Screening Programme, 2006.
4. Cancer Research UK website. UK Breast Cancer Incidence Statistics. London: Cancer Research UK, 2006. Available at: http://info.cancerresearchuk.org/cancerstats/types/breast/incidence/#age (last accessed 11 June 2006).
5. NHS Breast Screening Programme. *Building on Experience. Breast Cancer Screening Programme Annual Review 2002.* Sheffield: NHS Cancer Screening Programmes, 2002.

Lung cancer

STEPHEN SPIRO

Epidemiology of lung cancer

Lung cancer is extraordinarily common, appallingly difficult to treat and yet does not currently have a screening programme. It is the cause of death in 21% of men and 11% of women who die of cancer. The demography is changing: lung cancer was predominantly a disease of men, but small cell lung cancer, which constitutes around 20% of lung cancers, is now a disease of equal sex incidence. The combined deaths from all other common cancers – colorectal, breast, pancreatic and prostate – do not equal the number of people who die of lung cancer per year (Table 1). Figure 1 illustrates that because lung cancer is so lethal (with a median survival of about 8 months), the annual incidence is almost equal to the annual mortality. Trends in incidence and mortality parallel each other in men and in women; however, the incidence in men is decreasing with mortality as a direct result of smoking cessation, while in women, who are not stopping smoking in the numbers seen in men, the incidence and mortality is continuing to rise and will likely reach epidemic proportions. Screening or a new approach to treatment is desperately needed, as survival figures emphasize (Figure 2). Over the past 30 years, the number of people still alive 1 year after diagnosis has increased, probably because of the advent of chemotherapy rather than surgery, as 5-year survival, on which surgery has the most impact, has hardly improved over the last 20 years.

The reason for the failures in patients with lung cancer is that it has no particular disease-specific symptoms except for haemoptysis. GPs see only 1.5 new cases of lung cancer per year, and it is extremely difficult for them to differentiate patients with localized symptoms of lung cancer (haemoptysis, wheeze, cough or persistent respiratory infection) or symptoms that might develop into lung cancer from the hundreds of benign cases of cough, wheeze and chest infection. As with many solid tumours, when the disease presents to consultants, the tumour will be 3–4 cm in diameter, which is almost at the end of the natural history of the disease. Lung cancer can be detected on chest X-ray when the tumour reaches about 1 cm in diameter, but in 90% of patients diagnosed with a tumour 3–4 cm in size, a visible abnormality on previous chest X-rays will have been missed. The idea behind chest X-rays and, now, spiral

Table 1 Cancer statistics in 2003

Primary site	No. of new cases	No. of deaths	5-year survival rate (%)	
			1974–76	1992–78
Lung	171 900	157 200	12	15
Colorectum	147 500	57 100	50	62
Breast	212 600	40 200	75	86
Pancreas	30 700	30 000	3	4
Prostate	220 900	28 900	67	97

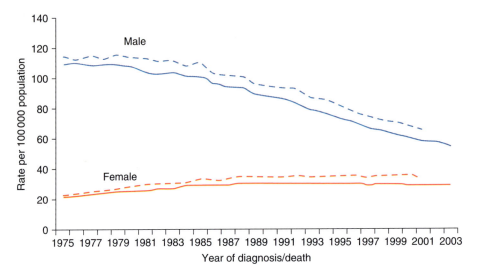

Figure 1
Incidence (_ _ _ _) and mortality (_____) of lung cancer in the UK, 1975–2003.

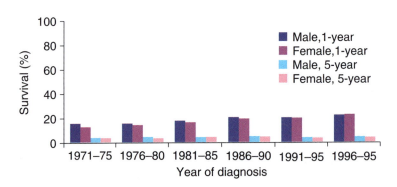

Figure 2
Relative survival from lung cancer in patients diagnosed in England and Wales, 1971–99.

and helical low-dose computed tomography (CT) is to identify solid tumours when they are much smaller, but halfway through the life of these tumours (20 volume-doubling times), they are just 1 mm in size and thus extremely hard to detect. The average size of tumours identified in published large hypothesis-generating studies using low-dose spiral CT is 15 mm.

Early studies of screening

Screening with an annual chest X-ray with or without sputum cytology was investigated extensively between the 1950s and 1970s. Studies that compared screening with no screening in similar control populations all showed increased detection of lung cancers and surgery in the active arm; however, the number of cases of advanced disease and the number of deaths were unaffected.[1-3] Contamination, as a result of people in the control group having chest X-rays outside the study, was a problem, as described for prostate cancer in Dr Boyle's chapter. In the Mayo Lung Project, for example, 55% of controls had chest X-rays, which makes the results difficult to interpret.[1] As a result, the concept of screening was abandoned in the mid-1970s.

Studies of low-dose spiral CT screening

The only current, reasonably available test likely to have any importance for screening is low-dose spiral CT. Some randomized studies are underway, but as they are unlikely to be published for several years, hypothesis-generating studies provide the only current results. The hypothesis in all such studies is that screening in asymptomatic high-risk individuals will identify early lung cancers (those at stage T1 in the TNM classification), which have a current 70% chance of cure. The Japanese Health Volunteer Population study included 1369 people (82% men) older than 50 years with a smoking history of more than 20 pack-years.[4] This type of population was chosen to increase the prevalence and, to some extent, the incidence yield of cancers. The patients underwent CT every 6 months. Screening at initial CT identified 15 cases (0.43%), with 14 of these being stage I with a mean diameter of 16 mm. Importantly, however, 11.4% of the scans were abnormal and needed further assessment.

The first published study arose from Claudia Henschke and the Early Lung Cancer Action Project (ELCAP) in New York.[5] It involved a high-risk population of 1000 volunteers older than 60 years, who had a smoking history of 45 pack-years and a life expectancy longer than 5 years (to ensure they were fit enough to undergo thoracotomy if cancer was identified). Each volunteer had a chest X-ray followed by low-dose CT, which identified about four times more cancers than chest X-ray: 223 versus 68 non-calcified nodules. The fact that there are four possible cell types (including large cell undifferentiated tumours) complicates the situation. Small cell lung cancer is so aggressive that it is very unlikely to be identified in an asymptomatic screen, and, indeed, most screening studies have failed to pick up this type of cancer. Squamous cell lung cancer, which is still the most common type in the UK, tends to be a central airway disease; it presents with haemoptysis and other similar symptoms and is rarely identified through CT. CT thus tends to isolate peripheral intrapulmonary tumours, which are almost always adenocarcinomas. This was reflected by the results of the study in New York: 27 of the 28 non-calcified nodules that were biopsied were cancerous, with 18 being identified as adenocarcinomas and 1 as a small cell lung cancer. Overall, the study had a high yield of stage I cancers and 26 of the 27 cancers were resectable (only 4 of which were visible on chest X-rays). The prevalence in this study was 2.7%.

A similar study from the Mayo Clinic took place in the middle of a region of the USA with a high incidence of histoplasmosis, coccidiomycosis and tuberculosis.[6] The study included 1520 people older than 50 years with a smoking history of at least 20 pack-years. Each patient had one prevalence screen and three annual incidence CT scans. The results from the prevalence screen were fairly similar to those from the other hypothesis studies, with 22 cancers being identified. The incidence screens in 1464 people found only three more cancers, which is in line with expectations. Overall, most were adenocarcinomas ($n=15$), six were squamous cell carcinomas, three were small cell cancers and one was a large cell cancer; 13 (60%) were at stage I. The problem with this study, as is often the case in CT screening, was the incidence of non-calcified nodules (2244 in 1000 patients), which accounted for a 98% incidence of false-positive findings because of the background of granulomatous disease. All radiologists involved in screening must follow careful algorithms to prevent people unnecessarily undergoing thoracotomy.

Overall, hypothesis studies of screening suggest that a high number of stage I cancers can be identified, but whether identifying cancers of this size will affect mortality is not yet known.

Randomized controlled studies of screening

Several randomized controlled studies of screening are underway in the USA and Europe. The largest is the National Lung Screening Trial (NLST) in the USA, which is part of the Prostate, Lung, Colorectal and Ovarian (PLCO) cancer trial. The 50 000 patients are smokers or former smokers aged 55–74 years with a smoking history of at least 30 pack-years. Patients are randomized to low-dose fast spiral CT or chest X-ray and undergo a prevalence screen, three annual incidence screens and 5-year follow-up. The results are likely to be reported in about 2011, but the approach is extremely expensive, with this study costing more than $200m (equivalent to £102m). In addition, the contamination may be very high, as high-resolution CT costs only about $200 in the USA and many patients randomized to receive chest X-rays in the study may be disappointed and seek CT elsewhere.

Combined analyses of studies on screening

Two papers have contrasting views on screening. The ELCAP investigators[7] analysed the results from several non-randomized studies across the world. The analysis included 31 567 individuals gathered over a 12-year period, who had a median age of 61 (range 40–85) years and a median smoking history of 30 (0–141) pack-years. Prevalence screens picked up 4186 (13%) nodules and incidence screens identified a further 1460 (5%). Of the small proportion of 535 biopsied nodules, 484 people received a diagnosis of cancer, with a very high proportion of stage I cancer, as is desired in a useful screening test for lung cancer. The authors concluded that if the results from these non-randomized data (Figure 3) are proved to be accurate and sustainable, screening will be worthwhile.

Bach et al[8] reviewed three hypothesis-generating studies (from Milan, the Mayo Clinic and Florida) that aimed to confirm whether or not screening increases the frequency of diagnosis and resection and reduces the risk of diagnosis of advanced disease or death. Overall, the analysis included 3246 asymptomatic current or ex-smokers from three centres, with a median follow-up of 3.9 years. The outcome measure was comparison of observations in studies with outcomes predicted in a well-validated model that takes into account individual risk factors. In the 3200 people screened, 144 cases of lung cancer were observed compared with 44 expected (relative risk 3.2; $p < 0.001$). The number of patients who underwent resection was about 10-fold higher than expected (109 vs 10.9; relative risk 10.0; $p < 0.001$), but there was no decline in the number of patients with advanced disease compared with the predicted number (42 observed vs 33 predicted) or the numbers of deaths (38 vs 38.8) (Figure 4).

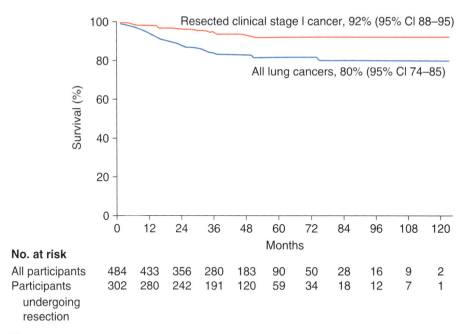

Figure 3
Kaplan-Meier survival curves for 484 participants with lung cancer and 302 participants with clinical stage I cancer resected within 1 month after diagnosis. Reproduced with permission from the International Early Lung Cancer Action Program Investigators.[7]

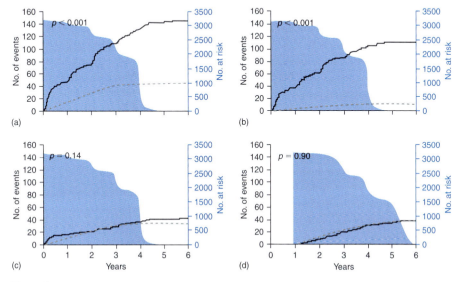

Figure 4
Combined diagnosis of lung cancer (a), surgical resections (b), diagnoses of advanced lung cancer (c) and deaths (d) from three studies. The curves show the numbers of events (_____, observed; _ _ _ _ _, predicted) and the shaded areas show the numbers at risk. Adapted from Bach et al.[8]

The group concluded that screening identifies more cases but does not reduce the numbers of advanced cases or deaths.

Bach et al[8] noted that the studies analysed have limitations: they are small and preliminary, and, unlike large trials in cervical and colon cancer that compare screened and unscreened populations, the comparator is an individual risk-factor predictive model. Some of the cases that contributed to the threefold increase in diagnoses of lung cancer through screening may not have progressed to clinical detection; however, others would have progressed to cause death if left untreated, and detection of these would justify screening, which mainly identifies a cohort of slowly growing tumours with low propensity to metastasize

Squamous cell carcinoma

In the UK, squamous cell cancer is the most common lung cancer seen at bronchoscopy. Squamous cell carcinomas evolve from epithelial abnormalities through low-grade abnormalities (mild and moderate dysplasia) then high-grade abnormalities (severe dysplasia and carcinoma in situ) until they finally become invasive cancers. Not all abnormalities produce carcinomas: carcinoma in situ disappears in some series, progresses in others and is stable in the remainder.

The London Lung Cancer Group has received funding to investigate screening in 1300 individuals at high risk – middle-aged people with mild and moderate chronic obstructive pulmonary disease (COPD), a heavy smoking history, or head and neck cancer. People allocated to a control group will undergo no screening, so that any cancers detected will be identified solely through general practice. The surveillance arm will have an annual sputum screen and surveillance CT and bronchoscopy as necessary for 5 years. The study will investigate whether sputum cytology can identify early mucosal changes and whether autofluorescence bronchoscopy can be used to detect dysplasia, carcinoma in situ and invasive cancer in patients with abnormalities in sputum cytology. It will also aim to determine whether or not dysplasia and carcinoma in situ always develop into invasive cancer and whether or not CT can offer further screening benefits in this population. The study will also compare the stage of cancers at diagnosis in the control and surveillance groups. It is hoped that the study will provide another approach to determine if yearly surveillance identifies a substantial number of lung cancers at an early stage, to determine if there is a more sensitive test than sputum cytology to look at the malignant potential of preinvasive lesions and to determine the level of compliance with annual screening.

Conclusion

Little evidence supports screening with chest X-rays. CT undoubtedly identifies more early cancers, particularly in populations of older predominantly male heavy smokers with reduced FEV_1 (forced expiratory volume in 1 second). No randomized trials are available. The issue of a high prevalence of benign non-calcifying nodules in centres that enter patients into studies needs to be resolved. Finally, views on whether or not CT screening will affect mortality are conflicting. Lung cancer is an extremely important cancer, but its regular treatment, apart from surgery, is very inadequate, and many doctors hope, therefore, that screening will be useful – but it may still be some time before that is the case.

References

1. Fontana R, Sanderson DR, Woolner LB et al. Lung cancer screening: the Mayo Program. *J Occup Med* 1986; **28**: 746–50.

2. Kubik A, Polak J. Lung cancer detection: results of a randomized prospective study in Czechoslovakia. *Cancer* 1986; **57**: 2428–37.

3. Melamed MR, Flehinger RB, Heelan RT et al. Screening for early lung cancer: results of the Memorial Sloan-Kettering study in New York. *Chest* 1984; **86**: 44–53.

4. Kaneko M, Eguchi K, Ohmatsu H et al. Peripheral lung cancer: screening and detention with low dose spiral CT versus radiography. *Radiology* 1996; **201**: 798–802.

5. Henschke CI, McCauley DI, Yankelevitz DF et al. Early Lung Cancer Action Project: overall design and findings from baseline screening. *Lancet* 1999; **354**: 99–105.

6. Swensen SJ, Jett JR, Hartman TE et al. Lung cancer screening with CT: Mayo Clinic experience. *Radiology* 2003; **226**: 756–61.

7. The International Early Lung Cancer Action Program Investigators. Survival of patients with stage I lung cancer detected on CT screening. *N Engl J Med* 2006; **355**: 1763–71.

8. Bach PB, Jett JR, Pastorino U et al. Computed tomography screening and lung cancer outcomes. *JAMA* 2007; **297**: 953–61.

Cancer in children

ALAN CRAFT

Introduction

Cancer in childhood is very rare compared with cancer in adults. Overall, childhood cancers account for only 0.5% of all malignancies, they occur in about 1 in 10 000 children per year, and 1 in 600 children will have cancer at some time during the first 15 years of their life. Childhood cancers are also usually more responsive to treatment than cancers in adults, and most children can be cured of their cancer, although at an average cost of £80 000–100 000. Children who are cured live a long time, however – perhaps another 70 or 80 years – so the annual cost per year saved is around £1000–2000, which makes the treatment of childhood cancer cost-effective.

Childhood cancer takes a variety of forms: one-third of cases are leukaemias, one-fifth are brain tumours and the remainder are a variety of other organ-based tumours (Box 1). The cause of most childhood cancers is unknown. Genetics may account for a small but increasingly recognized proportion of cases and may be a more common cause than currently realized. Environmental factors – in which children are exposed to a carcinogen – are probably very rare. Such exposure is most likely to occur in utero, and, indeed, some evidence suggests that the food that mothers eat during pregnancy can influence the development of some forms of childhood cancer: for example, consumption of large amounts of broccoli, which contains high levels of topoisomerase II inhibitors, has been linked with an increased incidence of infant leukaemia. A variety of products inhibit topoisomerase II, including red wine. Overall, however, the aetiology of childhood cancer is probably multifactorial.

Box 1 Childhood malignancies

- Bone tumours
- Epithelial tumours
- Germ cell tumours
- Leukaemias (34%)
- Liver tumours
- Lymphomas
- Neuroblastoma
- Renal tumours
- Retinoblastoma
- Sarcomas
- Central nervous system tumours (20%)
- Miscellaneous

Fortunately, survival from childhood cancer is improving, with 1 in every 900 young adults in the population being a survivor of childhood cancer and its treatment. Indeed, every 5-year period from 1962 has seen a progressive increase in survival, which still seems to be increasing, albeit at a slower rate than in earlier years.

Most childhood cancer is treatable. On the other hand, the prospects for prevention are not encouraging. For the few cancers that may have a genetic basis, prenatal diagnosis may be possible. However, the most important factor in prevention is perhaps to allow children to get dirty – the incidence of leukaemia has increased significantly over the last 30–40 years, almost certainly as a result of increased cleanliness in the population. Indeed, the more 'advanced' a society, the higher the rate of acute lymphoblastic leukaemia in childhood.

Conditions eligible for screening should be serious, have a detectable preclinical phase and be more treatable in the preclinical phase than in later stages. Screening can be population-based or targeted. For childhood cancer, early detection must be proved to be possible, and a simple screening test with high sensitivity and specificity is needed. There must be clear evidence that early detection makes a difference and that there is progression from an early to a late state – that is, from a good to a bad prognosis. Neuroblastoma fulfils all of these criteria.

Neuroblastoma

Neuroblastoma is the most common extracranial solid tumour in children. There are about 120 cases in the UK each year, and it represents about one-tenth of all childhood malignancies. Across Europe, probably around 600 children have neuroblastoma, with about 40 of these being high-risk cases that are associated with poor survival compared with the other childhood cancers. High-risk neuroblastoma is one of the major reasons children still die of childhood cancer and one of the most common causes of death in children if accidents and congenital abnormalities are excluded.

Survival from neuroblastoma seems to be influenced by age and stage (Figure 1). The younger a patient, the more likely it is that they are in stage I rather than stage IV. As survival is better for stage I neuroblastoma and for children of younger age, neuroblastoma seems to present the ideal situation for screening.

There is urinary excretion of diagnostic markers in more than 95% of patients with neuroblastoma: catecholamine metabolites in urine can be identified relatively easily with high-performance liquid chromatography (HPLC) or similar techniques. Tadashi Sawada from Kyoto, Japan pioneered screening using this approach from the early 1970s onwards. In 1988, a group led by his colleague Takeo Takeda published a paper that compared the effect of mass screening in Sapporo City on Hokkaido (the northern island of Japan) with no screening on the rest of Hokkaido by considering survival from neuroblastoma in the screened and unscreened areas.[2] Figure 2 shows that there was no change in survival for Hokkaido excluding Sapporo City, but a dramatic increase in survival for Sapporo City during the 3 years in which screening was undertaken. On the basis of these results, Sawada and colleagues persuaded the Japanese government to mandate neuroblastoma screening for the whole of the Japanese population. For the last 25 years, every Japanese baby has been offered screening at the age of 6 months, and around 25 million children have been screened to date.

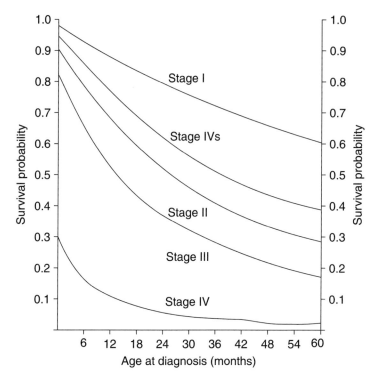

Figure 1

Survival related to stage and age in 246 cases of neuroblastoma. Adapted with permission from Breslow and McCann.[1]

In the 1980s, pilot/feasibility studies in the North of England evaluated whether this apparent improvement in survival was true. We tested for catecholamines in urine collected from babies aged 6 months. From 10 000 screened children, we found four babies with neuroblastoma – all of whom were successfully treated surgically and are alive today. During this period, however, understanding of the biology of neuroblastoma was improving and it was beginning to be recognized that there were 'good' and 'bad' neuroblastomas and that some regressed spontaneously. It also became apparent that the Japanese screening process was actually identifying children with conditions other than neuroblastoma. We concluded that screening was practical, feasible and acceptable to parents, who were very keen to have their babies screened for cancer, but that it was very important to emphasize to parents that the children were not being screened for all forms of cancer.[3] We also concluded that a large randomized controlled trial with mortality from neuroblastoma as the only major endpoint was needed. A great deal of time and effort was spent designing a huge national trial, which was expected to prove that neuroblastoma screening did not work, but funding was eventually declined by the UK Medical Research Council on the basis that the study was unlikely to improve survival for children.

Researchers in Canada and Germany, however, were able to obtain funding from national authorities for major studies of screening. Woods et al[4] investigated screening in the province

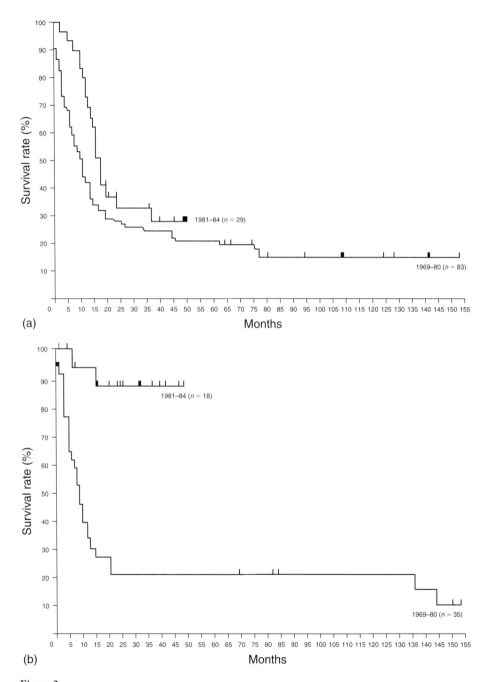

Figure 2
Survival curves in Hokkaido Prefecture (excluding Sapporo City) (a) and in Sapporo City (b) to 31 March 1986.
Screening was undertaken in Sapporo City between 1981 and 1984. Reproduced with permission from Nishi et al.[2]

of Quebec. Comparison of the standardized mortality rate (SMR) before and after screening in Quebec showed a slight increase in mortality after screening, which suggested that screening does not work. A comparison of SMRs showed no difference between Quebec and the rest of Canada. Finally, a comparison of the number of deaths expected in Quebec City on the basis of contemporaneously observed numbers in four control areas showed that Quebec had 22 cases when 20 would have been expected. Overall, therefore, screening did not seem to save lives. Researchers in Germany compared screening of babies aged 1 year in one half of Germany with no screening in the other half of the country.[5] The incidence of neuroblastoma doubled because screening picked up non-serious neuroblastomas, but the mortality per 100 000 did not differ between the screened and non-screened areas. The conclusion is that screening *does* detect tumours – but it probably detects tumours that would otherwise spontaneously regress.

Mortality from neuroblastoma thus is not decreased by screening, but the morbidity associated with screening in Japan is quite substantial. Around 1–2% of children who screened positive in Japan died during surgery to remove neuroblastomas that would have regressed spontaneously. A huge amount of time and effort is being exerted in Japan to withdraw the neuroblastoma screening programme, which is currently running in about half of the country, but with no real benefit for children.

The overall conclusion is that neuroblastoma screening does not work because molecular and genetic evidence confirms that the term encompasses at least three diseases:

- type I neuroblastoma, which involves no abnormalities of the genetic profile or chromosomes and has a 95% survival rate
- type II neuroblastoma, which involves abnormalities of chromosomes 11q, 3p and 14q that result in poorly differentiated tumours and a survival rate of 30%
- type III neuroblastoma, which involves chromosome 17q and *MYCN* abnormalities that result in very poorly differentiated tumours and a survival rate of just 15%

Wilms' tumours

Certain conditions, such as aniridia, hemihypertrophy and Beckwith–Wiedemann syndrome, predispose to childhood cancers, particular to Wilms' tumour. The birth incidences are estimated to be 1 in 10 000 for Wilms' tumour, 1 in 50 000 for aniridia, 1 in 17 000 for Beckwith–Wiedemann syndrome and around 1 in 53 000 for hemihypertrophy.[6] The incidence of these three predisposing conditions in Wilms' tumour is actually very low: 4.2–5.5% of patients with Wilms' tumours have aniridia, 0.8–1.9% have Beckwith–Wiedemann syndrome and 0.8–1.9% have hemihypertrophy. As most hemihypertrophies are not diagnosed until a child develops a Wilms' tumour, however, hemihypertrophies are not an appropriate target for screening.

We reviewed all cases of these conditions identified by screening in the National Childhood Register from Oxford and found no real evidence of a benefit from screening. As a result, we recommended teaching parents manual palpation of the abdomen. If necessary, we advocated screening with abdominal ultrasound every 3–4 months: Wilms' tumours grow rapidly, with a doubling time of 12–17 days, and this time period represents the window of opportunity for screening between the size at which the tumour can be diagnosed on ultrasound (about 1 cm^3) and the time of usual presentation (about 500 g).

Published guidance for surveillance for Wilms' tumours in high-risk populations concludes that the risks and benefits are finely balanced and that no clear evidence shows a reduction of mortality or morbidity.[7] The guidelines recommend that surveillance should be offered for children with a >5% risk of Wilms' tumour, using renal ultrasound every 3–4 months up to the age of 5 years (or 7 years in high-risk conditions, such as Beckwith–Wiedemann syndrome). This recommendation is based largely on that fact that once people know their baby is prone to cancer, they want a proactive approach, and as the numbers are fairly small, it is probably worth the effort for the sake of the parents.

Routine surveillance of children

Recognition that comparison of survival for adults with cancer in the UK with that in Europe showed the UK to be doing less well led to the National Cancer Plan. Recent publications comparing the survival of children with cancer across European countries have also shown an inferior outcome for the UK. In a recent presentation, Katherine Pritchard-Jones noted the need for access to high-quality population-based cancer registries, but highlighted that variations in national laws, systems and resources creates potential for 'significant' biases that must be considered in interpretation of any comparisons of different registry datasets.[8]

A large study undertaken in various countries, some with population-based registries and others with regional coverage, compared 5-year survival rates for childhood cancer.[10] The overall survival rate for the UK is 71%, which is lower than that in countries in the north (77%), south (72%) and west (75%) of Europe. These data correlate with findings from the Eurocare study,[11] which also showed 71% survival at 5 years in the UK, compared with higher survival rates elsewhere in Europe (76% for Germany, 75% for Norway, 79% for Sweden and 73% for France).

The UK's record for Wilms' tumour is significantly worse than that in Germany and the Scandinavian countries, probably for a number of reasons. Lack of referral to specialist centres cannot be a reason, because the number of children referred to specialist centres in the UK has increased rapidly over the last 15 years, with 99% of children with Wilms' tumour being treated in specialist centres. It is possible, however, that we are not using the best treatment or that we have a nihilistic approach to the treatment of relapse. This situation will hopefully improve now that guidance from the National Institute for Health and Clinical Excellence (NICE) is available and doctors in the UK are participating in international and European studies. Other reasons may include a difference in the extent of disease at presentation in the UK compared with continental Europe, which might be affected by differences in the mode of primary care for children. Furthermore, clinicians and parents in the UK might have a less-demanding approach to initial treatment and treatment of relapse.

To elucidate the reasons behind the poor results in the UK, we have undertaken a study to compare approaches in the UK with those in Germany, which seems to have an 8% better chance of survival than the UK. In Germany, children undergo extensive preventive medical examinations during the first 15 years of life (unpublished data, 2007). In the UK, for what seem to be reasons of cost-effectiveness, children are examined at birth and some also during the first year of life, most often by health visitors rather than GPs. All primary care paediatricians in Germany have ultrasound machines in their consulting rooms, which means that most children will have office ultrasound during preventive medical examinations. Data from Germany show that Wilms' tumour was diagnosed in 67% of children as a result of symptoms, while 27% of children diagnosed had no tumour-related symptoms or no symptoms at all and were identified during preventive medical examinations. Importantly, relapse-free survival rates were higher in those with no tumour-related symptoms, which suggests that screening allowed earlier diagnosis of Wilms' tumours.

In the Royal Marsden Hospital in London, 86% of Wilms' tumours are identified as a result of the presence of tumour-related symptoms, with only 4% of tumours being diagnosed incidentally. The situation is worse in the northern region of England, where none of the last 103 Wilms' tumours diagnosed between 1978 and 2006 was diagnosed incidentally during a health check, and 100 were found because of the symptoms and signs of this particular tumour. This suggests that universal screening for Wilms' tumour in primary care may lead to an earlier diagnosis and increased survival. As 100 000 children need to be screened to find one Wilms' tumour, however, routine surveillance is probably not economically worthwhile.

Conclusion

Neuroblastoma screening is not worthwhile. Targeted screening for high-risk populations is probably not worthwhile economically, but is important for parents. It is therefore vitally important that treatments for childhood cancers be improved, because prevention and screening will not have a major impact at present.

References

1. Breslow N, McCann B. Statistical estimation of prognosis for children with neuroblastoma. *Cancer Res* 1971; **31**: 2098–103.
2. Nishi M, Miyake H, Takeda T et al. Effects of the mass screening of neuroblastoma in Sapporo City. *Cancer* 1987; **60**: 433–6.
3. Parker L, Craft AW, Dale G et al. Screening for neuroblastoma in the north of England. *BMJ* 1992; **305**: 1260–3.
4. Woods WG, Gao RN, Shuster JJ et al. Screening of infants and mortality due to neuroblastoma. *N Engl J Med* 2002; **346**: 1041–6.
5. Schilling FH, Spix C, Berthold F et al. Neuroblastoma screening at one year of age. *N Engl J Med* 2002; **346**: 1047–53.
6. Craft AW, Parker L, Stiller C, Cole M. Screening for Wilms' tumour in patients with aniridia, Beckwith syndrome, or hemihypertrophy. *Med Pediatr Oncol* 1995; **24**: 231–4.
7. Scott RH, Walker L, Olsen ØE et al. Surveillance for Wilms tumour in at-risk children: pragmatic recommendations for best practice. *Arch Dis Child* 2006; **91**: 995–9.
8. Pritchard-Jones K. Survival of children with cancer in the UK in comparison with the rest of Europe: Do we have a problem? Abstract presented at the 11th Spring Meeting of the Royal College of Paediatrics and Child Health, York, UK, 26–29 March 2007.
9. Pritchard-Jones K, Kaatsch P, Steliarova-Foucher E et al. Cancer in children and adolescents in Europe: developments over 20 years and future challenges. *Eur J Cancer* 2006; **42**: 2183–90.
10. Sankila R, Martos Jiménez MC, Miljus D et al. Geographical comparison of cancer survival in European children (1988–1997): report from the Automated Childhood Cancer Information System Project. *Eur J Cancer* 2006; **42**: 1972–80.
11. Gatta G, Corazziari I, Magnani C et al. Childhood cancer survival in Europe. *Ann Oncol* 2003; **14**(Suppl 5): 119–27.

Discussion

WENDY ATKIN, PETER BOYLE, ALAN CRAFT, SILVIA FRANCESCHI, MICHAEL MICHELL, RICHARD PETO, STEPHEN SPIRO, ROBIN WILLIAMSON

Participant: Dr Boyle, a new breed of prostate markers such as *Pch3* in conjunction with prostate-specific antigen (PSA) seem to be emerging. Do you think they may be of more benefit in the future if they become low in cost and widely available?

Peter Boyle: A number of markers have emerged for prostate cancer, but after the promise of albumin urinary excretion (AUE) was not borne out, I am cautious about the utility of any markers until results from its implementation in large numbers of men are available. Overall, the development of new markers for prostate cancer has been disappointing: levels of PSA evolved into age-specific PSA, which became free and complexed PSA, and finally PSA velocity, which is still not ideal.

Richard Peto: Was the lifetime risk you discussed adjusted in some way for the fact that life expectancy is increasing?

Peter Boyle: The data were not standardized but were taken directly from data available from the cancer registry in the USA.

Participant: Benign prostate hyperplasia (BPH) and haematuria are the main drivers for men to request PSA tests. Do you think the average doctor would rely solely on a PSA test or would be seeking other well-known symptoms of BPH?

Peter Boyle: It is much easier to diagnose BPH than prostate cancer, as the International Prostate Symptom Score (IPSS) questionnaire and the American Urological Association's Symptom Index can be used to diagnose it without the need for any test. Furthermore, digital rectal examination by an experienced urologist has an almost 85% correlation with prostate volume as assessed by the PSA test. The PSA test thus is not an absolute necessity even in men who are complaining of urological symptoms compatible with BPH, as other methods of diagnosis are effective.

Silvia Franceschi: Professor Atkin, do you have any explanations for the difference in incidence of colorectal cancers in the proximal and distal parts of the colon and the peak age of incidence for distal carcinomas?

Wendy Atkin: Screening and polyp removal is probably responsible for the fall in incidence of distal colorectal cancer. Why this has not happened yet in the proximal colon is unclear. It may be due to technical failure in the endoscope reaching the caecum or to failure to find proximal polyps. Alternatively, proximal colon cancers may have a different biology. For example, it is unclear why the incidence of distal adenomas peaks in middle age while proximal adenomas increase throughout life or peak later in life.

Participant: Dr Michell, you mentioned that an increase in the upper age for screening is being considered. What is the current self-referral rate for women older than 70 years, and will increasing the upper age limit encourage more older women to attend for screening?

Michael Michell: The number of women older than 70 years who attend for screening voluntarily is increasing dramatically, with women in their 80s and sometimes 90s attending. After the age of 70 years, many women believe that their risk decreases because they are no longer called for screening, and some work is attempting to counteract that misconception. Screening in women older than 70 years is attractive, as the sensitivity and specificity are high because mammograms from women of this age group are easier to read; furthermore, women in their 70s are becoming increasingly fit and could gain a lot from screening.

Participant: Should the age of screening be lowered to 40 years?

Michael Michell: Trials have been undertaken in the UK and other countries. Current evidence suggests that screening of women in their 40s probably works, but the effect on mortality from breast cancer in the UK is less pronounced than the effect on mortality in women aged from 50 years. The latest results show a non-significant decrease in mortality of about 17%. It is difficult to decide whether screening should be introduced in this age group, because they represent a difficult age group for screening: there are fewer cancers, screening must be undertaken yearly because of the increased number of rapidly growing cancers, and the specificity is lower, which means that the recall rate would be higher. On balance, screening in women in their 40s is probably not appropriate for the UK at present.

Richard Peto: If the age range is to be extended in either direction, it does not need to be rolled out rapidly, and any extension should therefore be undertaken in a way that would be randomly informative so that the results could guide the rest of the world for decades.

Robin Williamson: Why is there not more research into screening for lung cancer?

Stephen Spiro: Screening is very expensive and computed tomography (CT) screening is extremely expensive. Although a pilot was discussed, it has been difficult to obtain funding. Cancer Research UK has funded our screening study.

Robin Williamson: Should treatment be withheld from smokers, as has been suggested recently?

Stephen Spiro: Around 80% of people who smoke develop lung cancer and 20% of patients with lung cancer have never smoked. As increasing numbers of ex-smokers are now developing lung cancer, I believe that all patients with lung cancer deserve equal treatment, and I believe that science demands this.

Robin Williamson: Do your screening techniques pick up other useful information, such as early tuberculosis or fungal conditions that merit early treatment?

Stephen Spiro: Unfortunately, CT identifies many confounding conditions. Up to 20% of scans show abnormalities such as occasional lymphomas, lymphadenopathy of no or indeterminant cause, thoracic and abdominal aneurysms, and lumps on the kidneys. This can create unnecessary anxiety for some patients, who have to be told about an abnormality that is often benign, although diagnosis of aneurysms is helpful.

Wendy Atkin: As sputum can be collected so simply and non-invasively, have you tried to extract DNA from the sputum to look for molecular markers?

Stephen Spiro: That will form part of our study, but it is not as simple as it might seem. The study needs to include people fit enough to undergo pulmonary resection, which means their lung function cannot be too compromised. Unfortunately, however, only about one-quarter of people with mild and moderate chronic obstructive pulmonary disease produce sputum spontaneously, so sputum needs to be induced with free normal saline in a nebulizer.

Robin Williamson: Is smoking during pregnancy relevant to the incidence of childhood cancer?

Stephen Spiro: Studies show conflicting results, but, on balance, smoking in the pregnant mother probably does have an effect.

Alan Craft: The evidence is not 100% clear; however, there is some evidence that smoking marijuana during pregnancy has an association with brain cancers and leukaemia in children.

Participant: Is it possible to extract a way to categorize and identify cancers according to whether or not they progress from the large ongoing trials on prostate and lung cancer?

Peter Boyle: In major series, 4% of Gleason 6 tumours adopt an aggressive posture that involves biological recurrence, real recurrence or clinical recurrence in a reasonable period of time. It has not yet been possible, however, to separate aggressive and non-aggressive cancers in terms of cytology, but work is ongoing to try to identify other factors that influence the aggressiveness of a tumour as well as its tumour grade.

Robin Williamson: That also seems to have been a challenge in neuroblastoma. Professor Craft, is there now an easy way to separate good from bad cancers?

Alan Craft: Once a neuroblastoma has been diagnosed and biopsied, it can be classified as good-risk or as bad-risk, and the treatment can be stratified accordingly. Some low-risk tumours are left alone to regress naturally.

Wendy Atkin: The real challenge with screening for all disease is not to harm people by unnecessarily introducing them 'into the system'.

Robin Williamson: Around 4–5 years ago, during a debate on the value of screening, a lay advocate spoke against screening on the basis of the enormous amount of angst caused for women who had false positives and then had to be reassured. Is that still a problem for breast cancer screening?

Michael Michell: False positives are a very important issue for any screening programme. Overdiagnosis of cancer in the breast cancer screening programme is currently estimated to affect one in eight of cancers diagnosed – in other words, the cancer would not have become manifest in the woman's natural lifespan. We are very conscious of this issue and discuss it clearly in the information leaflet given to all women invited for screening. About 6–7% of women have shadows on mammograms that require recalls for repeat tests but are found to be totally benign, and we are aware that patients become very anxious as a result of recalls, but we do know that anxiety does not persist after the assessment is complete.

Stephen Spiro: Overdiagnosis is a real phenomenon in lung screening. We see a number of high-risk patients after resection who are referred because follow-up bronchoscopy shows carcinoma in situ or because indeterminate cells have been left on the resection margins. We now have follow-up in a considerable cohort of high-risk people, some of whom have developed a sixth episode of lung cancer. They do not all have the same cell type, however, and in some we have removed carcinoma in situ, some have received photodynamic therapy for invasive cancer and some have developed peripheral adenocarcinomas. The conclusion is that some patients have a predisposition, probably triggered by smoking, that produces field cancerization in most patients with lung cancer.

Robin Williamson: What is the incidence of metachronous colorectal cancer?

Wendy Atkin: The incidence is about 5% over 10–15 years. Overdiagnosis is much less of an issue for colorectal cancer because the colorectum is easily accessible and benign adenomas can be removed non-invasively. The major problem is the resultant cost of repeat colonoscopy, because adenomas tend to recur. Data from the USA suggest that one-third of people who attend screening ultimately are engaged in some kind of surveillance programme, so algorithms have been developed to keep people out of the system.

Robin Williamson: Is there a case for more extensive colonic resection in younger people because of the risk of metachronous cancer 10–15 years later?

Wendy Atkin: Extensive colonic resection is not generally appropriate, except for patients with a very high risk due to inheritance of a genetic predisposition.

Robin Williamson: Is the field defect described by Professor Spiro important in terms of cancers in the second breast or elsewhere in the irradiated breast?

Michael Michell: Field cancerization is an issue in breast cancer, although perhaps more so for in situ carcinoma, which accounts for 20% of detected cancers. As the natural history of in situ carcinoma is uncertain, the effect of its detection and treatment on breast cancer mortality remains the subject of ongoing study and debate.

Participant: In the future, are screening programmes likely to be helpful for cancers other than those discussed today?

Peter Boyle: Several trials are ongoing. The UK Collaborative Trial of Ovarian Cancer Screening (UKC-TOCS) has already recruited 200 000 women and has a good follow-up phase, but the results are not expected for some time. Smaller trials are ongoing around the world. Trials are investigating bladder cancer screening using a test for a combination of antibodies, and other innovative approaches are under investigation. Trials of gastric cancer screening have been reported in Japan, but methodological issues have made interpretation difficult and initial evaluations were not convincing. Screening for oesophageal cancer is not promising, although some ideas involving people swallowing string or cotton wool to bring up enough cells for analysis are under development. The only three screening programmes currently recommended by the European Commission are for breast cancer, cervical cancer and colorectal cancer

Participant: Can screening help in the early detection of oral cancer?

Peter Boyle: A study of three rounds of visual inspection of the mouth in 90 000 men from Trivandrum, the capital of the Kerala region of Southern India, reported a 40% decrease in mortality from oral cancer in a screening group compared with a control group. The result was very significant, with the highest decreases being seen in people with risk factors, particularly smoking and alcohol consumption. Such visual inspection by highly trained technicians thus does have an effect, and this has been rolled out to other parts of India, with the Indian government 2 years ago announcing the creation of 350 rural cancer centres in the next 10 years. These centres will feed into a major state cancer centre and will be equipped with a series of cobalt machines to facilitate cancer registration and look for opportunities for early detection, particularly of cancers of the mouth and cervix. Two large randomized trials of screening for cervical cancer in India and Africa using very low-technology visual inspection methods trials will report this year, but initial data suggest a reduction in mortality of at least 40%.

Leszek Borysiewicz: How do people feel about screening methods independent of the normal access to healthcare systems?

Wendy Atkin: Before the bowel cancer screening programme was introduced, a number of private healthcare companies were considering offering faecal occult blood testing at very low cost. I felt very strongly that if the companies are not prepared to undertake and pay for colonoscopies if the screening is positive, then they should not be offering such screening. The real costs of screening are the investigations, and it is irresponsible for private companies to impose this extra burden of investigations on the health service.

Stephen Spiro: Unfortunately, there are no very good predisposing markers in lung cancer, but private companies have set up CT and cardiac screens that show the lungs very nicely. In the UK, between 1 in 9 and 1 in 11 people will have a non-calcified nodule on those CTs. This causes a huge amount of anxiety, and the NHS often has to pick up the cost of follow-up now that radiologists have good management algorithms.

Michael Michell: The population's behaviour has changed completely over the last 20 years, with increased emphasis on breast awareness, better health education and better publicity about the screening programme. Fungating breast cancers, which were common 20 years ago, are now very rare, which is a good thing. On the other hand, symptomatic breast clinics in the UK are now facing a huge workload caused by the worried well. The most appropriate way to cope with this is not clear, because tests are very expensive and there is a grey area in which, rightly or wrongly, women in their 40s who attend a breast clinic will almost certainly receive a mammogram.

Peter Boyle: The fall of the Soviet Union led to a breakdown in family practice and prevention services, and the Russian government has been trying to restore these services. One of the consequences is that 80% of cases of cancer diagnosed in Russia have been at an advanced, uncurable stage. As a result, the Russian government took the initiative about a year ago to set up an early detection programme; this involved rapidly retraining 15 000 hospital doctors to become GPs in a series of factories and cooperatives throughout the former Soviet Union. In the first year, the doctors undertook clinical examination with minor biochemistry in 7.5 million Russians, with another eight million due to be examined this year. We are evaluating the programme to determine whether this approach will lead to a downstaging to help reduce the 80% rate of incurable cancers. Early indicators already suggest better rates in breast cancer, colorectal cancer and gastric cancer, with people being identified with symptoms but earlier in the disease process. The importance of such downstaging in rapidly reducing mortality in any country is often overlooked.

Participant: Quantum physics claims that merely observing a phenomenon alters the phenomenon itself. Is there any evidence that detecting a tumour and investigating it by biopsy or excision alters the behaviour of that tumour for the worse?

Michael Michell: Patients frequently and very sensibly ask this question when they are undergoing further tests and biopsies. I believe that any effect of percutaneous biopsy on the behaviour of breast cancers would have been observed by now, but there is no evidence of such an effect. Some excellent studies have histologically investigated tumours, the surrounding tissue and the track taken by the needle, and have shown that although the needle passing through a tumour displaces tumour cells, those cells seem to become non-viable without the potential for metastatic spread.

Alan Craft: Neuroblastomas are always examined very carefully, but the biopsy track is very important for any serious and malignant childhood cancer and is usually excised along with the tumour.

Peter Boyle: The only evidence for an issue with transrectal biopsy for prostate cancer was a very rare sarcoma that had seeded along the track of the biopsy.

Leszek Borysiewicz: In cervical cancer, evidence suggests that tumour biopsies are beneficial rather than detrimental.

Stephen Spiro: Investigation of mesothelioma involves a biopsy taken through the chest wall, and the incidence of tumour spread down the track is so high that patients routinely receive a single fraction of radiotherapy to the biopsy site. This is quite different to the situation with lung cancer, for which the risk is minimal.

Participant: Could stools be examined bacteriologically to investigate a link between bacterial populations and possible risks of cancer?

Wendy Atkin: A lot of work is ongoing in terms of analysis of bacterial flora. Research is already showing the complexity and stability of the flora, which seems to be established very early in life. Huge variations are seen, however, and it would be interesting to understand the bacterial origins, as much evidence suggests that something happens in adolescence to cause the onset of adenomas, particularly in patients with familial adenomatous polyposis. Understanding of colorectal cancer is really in its infancy.

Stephen Spiro: A paper in *The Lancet* 5–6 years ago reported on investigations of the volatile organic compounds in the breath that had identified 15–20 aromatic amines. The authors advocated testing for these compounds, and initial investigations seemed promising, but the research does not seem to have progressed any further.

The Jephcott Lecture

Cancer prevention: vaccine-based approaches

LESZEK BORYSIEWICZ

Cancer immunology

In 1943, Gross realized that carcinogens such as methylcholanthrene could induce sarcomas in mice.[1] Prehn and Main then showed that immunity to these tumours could be transferred from one mouse to another but that the antigens were tumour-specific:[2] that is, antibodies from a tumour in mouse A given to mouse B were effective only against tumour cells from mouse A. These data raised the possibility of inducing a immune response against tumours, in which the body recognizes tumour cells as foreign but does not recognize differences between different strains. The 1960s saw much research in this field, but the results are epitomized by Hewitt's conclusion: mouse tumours were insufficiently distinct to activate the immune system, making immunological intervention futile.[3] In the 1980s, tumours were recognized not to be passive partners but to be composed of active cells that grow and mutate constantly so that they are able to evade responses the host raises against them.

Vaccine-based approach to cancer prevention

Vaccines are the singularly most interesting and effective healthcare interventions – other than clean water and food supplies – to have made a difference in terms of the prevalence and incidence of disease. Over the past 20 years, major advances in molecular understanding of tumour biology and immunology have made novel approaches realistic: although the principles espoused in the 1940s and 1950s were absolutely correct, researchers were unable to move the concept into reality. The key has been the move away from the focus on antibodies as the main mediators of immunity to tumours and the recognition that the cellular component of the immune response eradicates cells, whereas antibodies work against particulate matter. Molecular techniques have also made identification of specific tumour antigens much easier. This has raised major debate about whether tumour vaccines should be therapeutic or prophylactic.

An effective vaccine against cancer has to recognize the cancer as foreign, generate appropriate protective immunity, home in on the site of the tumour, generate a long-lasting immunogenic response and prevent the tumour evading the generated response. An enormous explosion in the literature on tumour antigens has occurred. Many classification systems for tumour antigens are in use, but the most relevant recognizes two major types of 'foreignness' about a cancer cell. The first is a 'private' foreignness, in which tumour antigens are patient-specific; this means that one person's lung cancer is quite distinct antigenically from another person's lung cancer. To use an immunogenic approach with these antigens would require a personalized, and thus costly, approach to treatment or prevention, so the next step is to investigate a more general approach in which antigens might work against a specific tumour type. Among this group, viral antigens are particularly important.

Human papillomaviruses

Human papillomaviruses (HPV) are a large family of DNA viruses, with 80 types identified and some 200 more predicted to exist. They are exquisitely beautiful but present problems for virologists because they can be seen only by electron micrography and cannot be grown in in vitro systems. They infect skin and mucosal epithelial cells, and some cause warts, which are growth dislocations of epithelial cells.

The infectious cycle of these agents is well known, and their development and ability to replicate are closely tied to the biology of an epithelial surface (Figure 1). The virus particles enter the system through the basal layer, where they begin to express certain viral non-structural gene products. The virus replicates and sheds from the surface as the epithelial cells mature. Warts and other lesions caused by HPV thus shed virus externally rather than internally, which means that the only antigens regularly exposed to the immune system are a few internal gene products, as the virus capsid is released at the surface. As a result, the infected cells and viruses survive, and 10^4 virus particles can be released from a single cell.

The virus has adapted to life with humans. It replicates slowly so as not to alert the immune system to its presence, and its ultimate aim is not to kill the host but to shed. After the virus enters the basal layers, cervical intraepithelial neoplasia 1 (CIN1) may be observed; this simply reflects infection of the cervical cells with HPV and is benign, with good evidence suggesting that this dysplasia could be left alone. Clinical disease is present for around 9 months. Spontaneous clearance is invariable in the case of warts and can occur in people with genital infections with the cancer-related viruses although treatment is often advocated as there is a

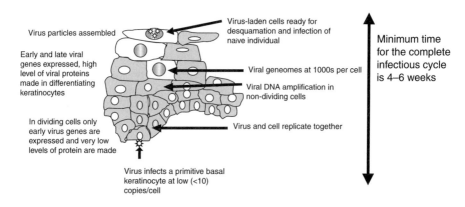

Figure 1

Infectious cycle of a human papillomavirus. (Adapted from Stanley MA. JNCI Monograph – Future Directions in Epidemiologic and Preventive Research on Human Papillomaviruses and Cancer 2003; 31: 117–24.)

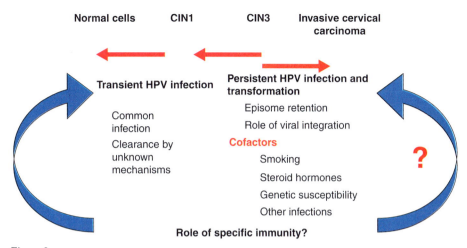

Figure 2
Development of cervical neoplasia.

low risk of persistence and later progression. The immune system seems to play a major role in mediating clearance, and normally the infection is cleared, with no long-term impact on the host. If the virus persists, however, dysplasia can progress and may eventually result in invasive cervical carcinoma (Figure 2), which is the second most common cancer in women worldwide, with 400 000 women presenting every year. Progression to invasive cervical carcinoma involves changes in the nature of the viral genome, as integration into the host genome occurs. Other cofactors also become important. Well-documented, observable and measurable rates of regression of the disease occur throughout the process at all stages as a result of the natural actions of the immune system, so it seems that cancer is the unintended, rare 'side-effect', particularly because of changes that occur in the virus–host interaction.

Approaches to vaccination

Therapeutic vaccination – preventing the transformation to cervical cancer

Infection with HPV is immunologically tractable because only two viral proteins of HPV – E6 and E7 – exist at the level of the basal cells. These proteins transform cells by interfering with cell growth by binding to tumour suppressor proteins (p53 and pRb), and inhibition of E6 and E7 reduces the growth potential of transformed cells. Studies suggest that only about eight of the 200 HPV types are likely to be oncogenic, with two types (HPV-16 and HPV-18) dominant across the world. This knowledge represented a breakthrough, as induction of an immune response against a common viral antigen that relates to just two proteins from two viruses (i.e. four proteins in total) is not inconceivable. This meant that it was possible to create a vector that could be used in humans once the site likely to induce oncogenic transformation was removed.

A vector was constructed and included in a vaccine virus that we tested in patients in South Wales in the first European study of a live recombinant agent against cancer.[4] Unfortunately, seven of the patients with late-stage cervical cancer died, but the vaccine was able to generate a transient cellular immune response. In one patient, who is still alive today, disease that had extended into the spinal cord regressed, although whether the vaccine was involved in this regression is uncertain. We also identified these HPV-specific T cells in higher frequencies at the sites of tumours. These cells were also identified only in patients with tumours, which suggests that local inoculation to these particular proteins occurs in the host in those with CIN3 or cancer.[5] Unfortunately, further phase I and phase II studies produced no evidence of a clinical effect, despite induction of the desired immune response.

A variety of reasons could explain this (Box 1). A team in Cardiff examined whether or not something happening in the tumour itself was stopping the vaccine being effective. Their work showed that although the vaccine generated a response quite easily, certain tumour cells (even though they carried the virus) were not able to process effectively the recognition signal seen by such cytotoxic T cells. Therefore, mutations in cancer cells, in the processing machinery, were sufficient to block an effective response.

Prophylactic vaccination – preventing infection with HPV

As the strains of virus that cause cancer worldwide are very stable, an alternative approach to preventing the transformation to cancer is to attempt to prevent HPV infection in the first place. Schiller and colleagues at the National Cancer Institute made a breakthrough in this area with a simple experiment in which the gene for the main capsid protein was expressed and released as a protein, which was folded into the shape of the virus particle. Importantly, the 'virus particle' contained no DNA, which meant that all of the oncogenic potential was

---

Box 1 Factors that limit the effectiveness of antitumour immunity
- Major histocompatibility complex
  - Haplotype
  - Altered expression
- Tolerance versus ignorance
- Tumour stroma
- Antigen and epitope loss variants
- Antigenic modulation
- Immune enhancement and blockade
- Immune suppression
  - Tumour inducers
  - Tumour burden
  - Treatment
  - Age

removed. Animal experiments showed that these virus-like particles (VLPs) were as immunogenic as the virus itself.

The first trial of a vaccine containing a VLP against HPV-16 was reported by Koutsky et al.[6] The study involved 2392 female students starting college. These women would be assumed to come into contact with many wild-type papillomaviruses, as the prevalence of HPV in the genital tracts of women aged 18 years in the USA is up to 20%. Indeed, within 9 months of the onset of sexual activity, most women have had exposure to an oncogenic type of this virus. Half of the women received the vaccine on three occasions and the other half received placebo. On initial follow-up at about 17.4 months, the women were analysed for the presence or absence of virus, and, remarkably, no persistent HPV infections were recorded in women who had been vaccinated compared with 41 cases in those who had received placebo. All 5 cases of HPV-related dysplasia occurred in the placebo group, with non-HPV-related changes seen in 22 women in each group. The study did have a number of limitations. The participants were very young, and the spontaneous rate of clearance would be expected to be high. The definition of persistence used – the presence of the same virus within 6 months – did not fulfil the purist definition of persistence. The follow-up period was very short, so that the decay of the antibody response was unknown. The design also failed to consider reinfection. Nevertheless, this study was a remarkable piece of work. Follow-up data confirm the promising findings of the early results: 5 years later, levels of apparently protective antibodies remain at the levels found after three immunizations, which suggests long-lived immunity (Koutsky, unpublished data, 2007).

Vaccination against one HPV strain will not protect against the other seven types of high-risk HPV, but Koutsky and colleagues found that it is possible to make and combine virus particles of different types (HPV-16, -18, -45, -31, -6 and -11) without inhibiting the production of antibodies against any of the individual types (Figure 3). In other words, multivalent vaccines are relatively simple to put together from a practical point of view and relatively easy to compile pharmacologically.

A plethora of studies have now been undertaken, and have confirmed that there are no significant adverse side-effects of multivalent vaccines.[7] As it will not be possible to prove an effect on cancer for around 50 years, dysplasia is used as a surrogate clinical endpoint. Studies have shown that some of the viruses are very closely related – for example, HPV-45 is very akin to HPV-18, and HPV-31 is very akin to HPV-16; for the first time, therefore, studies have hinted that cross-protection and cross-priming may be possible. Evidence also now suggests that the vaccine is probably ineffective in women already infected and thus only prevents primary infection. This means that vaccination must take place before the onset of sexual activity as there is no evidence of regression of any established disease or reduced transmission. The longest endpoints currently are follow-up at 5 years, so the long-term duration of protection remains uncertain although we should be optimistic based on comparable vaccines.

Combined approach to vaccination

The two approaches to vaccination – therapeutic and prophylactic – can be combined by adding the oncogenic protein and epitopes that the T cells see to the L-tail, which enables the

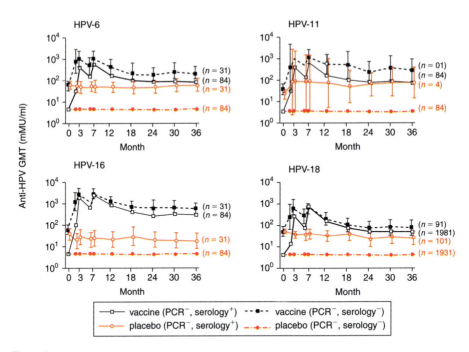

Figure 3

Levels of anti-HPV from a quadrivalent vaccine. Reproduced with permission from Koutsky and Harper.[7]

L1 virus capsid to cross-prime and develop cytotoxic T-cell responses. Studies are already showing promising results in this area, and VLPs could become important delivery systems for a whole range of T-cell-based vaccines.

Vaccination in practice

Vaccine candidates must meet certain criteria before they are introduced for widespread use. They must:[8]

- address the public health need and be a logical means of control
- have a sound scientific rationale
- have an expectation of safety
- have evidence of immunogenicity from animal studies
- be better than other alternative available measures
- be prepared in a practical and cost-effective formulation

We undertook a study to clarify the distribution of oncogenic subtypes in rural communities unperturbed by confounding variables such as HIV infection, in order to confirm that the vaccine would address the public health need and be a logical means of control. We identified 40 villages with good demographic characteristics in the Gambia and screened every woman (with the communities' consent) to try to establish the impact of an HPV-16/-18 vaccine on the natural incidence of infection. The cancer-causing strains still seemed to be HPV-16 and -18: although the population is Islamic and there is relatively limited exchange of partners, particularly in rural communities, 13.6% of the population was infected with these high-risk viruses. In the first 20 villages, we identified six new HPV types. African variants of HPV-16 and -18 are different to the circulating variants in Europe; such variants have also been found in Mozambique and other African countries. The relevance of this to the L1 protein is uncertain, but it could mean the need for different versions of multivalent HPV vaccines for different populations. The results confirm that the situation in the developing world may be some way removed from the reality in developed countries, and further studies of clinical effectiveness should be carried out in these high-risk communities.

Safety has been confirmed to 5 years to date. Animal studies of immunogenicity exist, but it is important to remember that papillomaviruses are totally species-specific and there is no model for genital infection.

The International Agency for Research on Cancer (IARC) has been investigating alternative control measures for the developing world. In Thailand and India, visual inspection of the cervix – perhaps the simplest form of screening imaginable – seemed to reduce the burden of disease by at least 40%. This approach makes women in developing countries more aware that this disease can kill, which is important, because cancer is a relatively novel phenomenon in many societies. Testing for papillomavirus could be an alternative approach to screening; however, it is still quite an expensive option and the cytological facilities in many developing countries would not be able to support the infrastructure needed to ensure that a programme is effective.

The vaccine formulation is certainly practical, but initial costs seem quite high, with a private price in Europe of €500–600 (£340–400) for a course of vaccinations. This would be very expensive for health ministers in developing countries, who might have $1.5 (£0.76) per year to spend on the health of an individual in a population. As two pharmaceutical companies are currently battling for the market share, market forces are likely to considerably drive down the price of the two current vaccinations, and social pressures from the World Health Organization and other organizations may encourage the companies to make the vaccinations available at a reasonable price in areas of high prevalence.

Vaccination in the developing world faces other obstacles. The Gambia has three ethnic languages, and there is no word for cancer: wasting disease and weight loss mean HIV or tuberculosis. This is despite the fact that the life expectancy has increased from 40 to 55 years and cancers are now emerging. Social change, education and empowerment of women will be needed to help them understand that postmenopausal bleeding is an indication of a disease and not the return of fertility and to ensure the successful implementation of vaccination or other strategies to prevent cervical cancer in developing countries. Studies in this setting thus are needed to confirm the effectiveness of this programme. Other issues that might block further development through studies in the developing world include:

- the Human Tissue Act, which makes it extremely difficult to transfer tissue samples for study

- the EU Clinical Trials Directive, when implemented in the EU; this directive blocks studies in developing countries and influences their acceptability in Europe
- cross-cultural ethical issues, which make it difficult to carry out initial studies in a developing country when they have not yet been studied in the developed world; this may be necessary because patient populations or numbers required to achieve the required power for a study may not be sufficient in the developed world, which thus requires trials to be undertaken in areas with a higher prevalence
- issues related to clinical trials in developing countries

Although these controls are in place for good reasons, they present major obstacles to the further development of vaccination through studies in developing countries. Studies in the developing world also introduce a range of potential ethical controversies related to HPV vaccination: the degree of conflict of interest of investigators and pharmaceutical companies, the nature and definition of effective and ethical best clinical care, the actions to be taken in respect of diseases other than cervical cancer discovered during screening of participants, the appropriate placebo (e.g. another vaccine such as rabies vaccine), good clinical practice in the study setting, and exposure of health inequalities. Indeed, the IARC has shown that, once the confounding variable of smoking is removed, cervical cancer is the one cancer that correlates with poverty regardless of the society.

Vaccination in the UK

Figure 4 illustrates the impact of the national call–recall system on the cytology programme in the UK.[9] The effectiveness of this programme apparently argues against the need for vaccination in the UK, but not all women attend for screening, and cervical cancer occurs in those women who do not attend. The long-term impact of the vaccination on mortality asso-

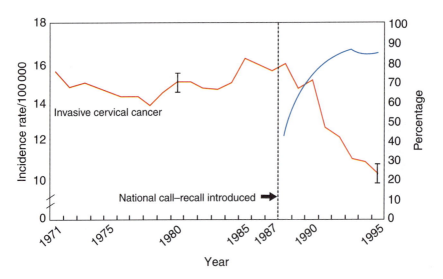

Figure 4

Age-standardized incidence of invasive cervical cancer and coverage of screening in England, 1971–95. Reproduced with permission from Castle et al.[9]

ciated with cervical cancer comes at a very high price in developed countries, such as the UK, because the screening system already picks up early disease and thus the vaccination will have little impact on mortality (Figure 5a). If the vaccination has only a 10-year effect and is not repeated, however, the impact on the disease will be reduced and vaccination will fail. Furthermore, vaccination against HPV-16 and -18 does not prevent all cases of cervical cancer. It thus is unlikely to be acceptable to stop screening when the vaccine programme is imple-

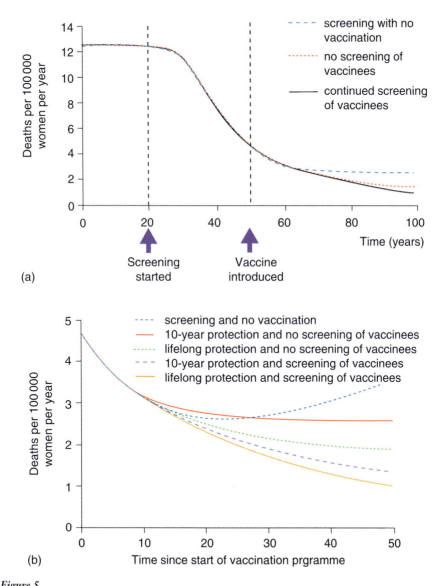

Figure 5

Mortality associated with cervical cancer (a) and impact of 10-year vaccine protection without boosters (b). Reproduced with permission from Garnett et al.[10]

101

mented. If the number of cases of cervical cancer is considered, however, 70% of cases of cervical cancer would be prevented over a 40-year period.

A number of factors will impact on the success and cost of the vaccination programme: degree of universal coverage, vaccination of men and women, catch-up programmes in people older than the age set for vaccination who are not yet sexually active, continued access to screening for those susceptible to disease and the behaviour of the viral population.

Conclusion

A vaccine-based approach to prevention of cervical cancer is now realistic, because the technology is available and we have a better understanding of pathogenicity and target identification. Vaccination could ultimately prevent the 25% attributable fraction of infection-related cancer that is particularly damaging in developing countries. The success of such a programme is constrained by the economics of delivering vaccination to a developing world at a high price and cost and with a delivery chain that ensures it is implemented. Furthermore, studies of the long-term impact are necessary and invaluable, but they require a long-term commitment towards funding that is difficult to find. Regulatory issues include the fact that cervical cancer has no animal model, which thus necessitates early studies in humans and raises political issues with respect to long-term investment and commitments in unstable government relations. This will require international, intergovernmental and academic–commercial partnerships that are also acceptable to local societies. If vaccination coverage falls below 70%, however, all investment by government for the public health issue will be a waste of time and money. As a result, economic, regulatory and political contexts will determine the success or otherwise of this programme.

References

1. Gross L. Intradermal Immunization of C3H mice against a sarcoma that originated in an animal of the same line. *Cancer Res* 1943; **3**: 326–33.
2. Prehn RT, Main JM. Immunity to methylcholanthrene-induced sarcomas. *J Natl Cancer Inst* 1957; **18**: 769–78.
3. Hewitt HB, Blake ER, Walder AS. A critique of the evidence for active host defence against cancer, based on personal studies of 27 murine tumours of spontaneous origin. *Br J Cancer* 1976; **33**: 241–59.
4. Borysiewicz LK, Fiander A, Nimako M et al. A recombinant vaccinia virus encoding human papillomavirus types 16 and 18, E6 and E7 proteins as immunotherapy for cervical cancer. *Lancet* 1996; **347**: 1523–7.
5. Evans EM, Man S, Evans AS, Borysiewicz LK. Infiltration of cervical cancer tissue with human papillomavirus-specific cytotoxic T-lymphocytes. *Cancer Res* 1997; **57**: 2943–50.
6. Koutsky LA, Ault KA, Wheeler CM et al. A controlled trial of a human papillomavirus type 16 vaccine. *N Engl J Med* 2002; **347**: 1645–51.
7. Koutsky LA, Harper DM. Current findings from prophylactic HPV vaccine trials. *Vaccine* 2006; **24**(Suppl 3): S114-21.
8. Tacket CO, Rennels MB, Mattheis MJ. Initial clinical evaluation of new vaccine candidates: phase 1 and 2 clinical trials of safety, immunogenicity, and preliminary efficacy. In: Levine MM, Woodrow GC, Kaper JB, Cobon GS, eds. *New Generation Vaccines: The Molecular Approach*. New York: Marcel Dekker, 1997.
9. Castle PE, Solomon D, Schiffman M, Wheeler CM. Human papillomavirus type 16 infections and 2-year absolute risk of cervical precancer in women with equivocal or mild cytologic abnormalities. *J Natl Cancer Inst* 2005; **97**: 1066–1071.
10. Garnett GP, Kim JJ, French K, Goldie SJ. Modelling the impact of HPV vaccines on cervical cancer and screening programmes. *Vaccine* 2006; **24**(Suppl 3): S178–86.

Discussion

Participant: At a recent meeting, researchers suggested that the incidence of cervical cancer is lower in France than in other countries. Could this be related to the natural history of the disease?

Leszek Borysiewicz: In France, many women are advised to visit a gynaecologist regularly, which effectively means that French women are screened on an almost annual basis. It is unclear whether this health-seeking behaviour in France has led to reduced levels of cervical cancer, but no evidence to my knowledge suggests a genetic difference in their predisposition to these agents, because the prevalence and incidence of infection are virtually the same in France as elsewhere in the world.

Participant: You mentioned a requirement for screening despite the apparent efficacy of the vaccine. Can you envisage a situation in which a good HPV screening approach will be completely eliminated by the effectiveness of the vaccine?

Leszek Borysiewicz: I believe that we overscreen for cervical cancer, as very little evidence suggests that screening is needed more than twice in a woman's sexually active life provided that HPV is screened for as well as cytology and the incidence of screening thus could be reduced quite dramatically. Debate surrounds the appropriate age at which screening should begin, with the Americans initiating screening at a far earlier age than is the case in the UK. Evidence for screening in women younger than 25 years is limited; although not screening women younger than 25 years in Holland would mean that a small number of cases of cervical cancer per annum would be missed. With the advent of the vaccine, access to the screening programme may need to more tightly controlled than is currently the case. The real benefit of the vaccine, however, will not be seen for another 40 years. Screening will still be necessary, because the vaccine does not cover all HPV types and there will, therefore, still be residual evidence of disease. The frequency of screening may need to reduced, but how acceptable closing down the screening programme is to its recipients is more likely to determine its survival than mathematical modelling. Overall, therefore, I believe that screening will continue. Importantly, however, the 20% of women who do not currently participate in the screening programme are also likely to avoid vaccination, and this above all must be addressed.

David Coggon: Does the strong socioeconomic gradient relate to exposure to infection, resistance to infection or a completely different factor?

Leszek Borysiewicz: There seems to be no obvious explanation, as all the simple confounders have been shown to have no effect. Studies in South America, for example, have shown that the number of sexual partners does not completely explain this phenomenon. Smoking also does not provide an explanation. It is likely that a number of factors are involved, and factors such as co-infection in resource-poor countries and hygiene are under consideration.

Index

Note: Page references in *italic* refer to tables or figures in the text